MILICA VL

HEALTHY BODY CLEANSE:

Gently Burn Body Fat and Lose Weight Naturally

Milica Vladova

"Healthy Body Cleanse: Gently Burn Body Fat and Lose Weight Naturally"

Copyright © 2016 by Militsa Vladova

All rights reserved.

FREE EBOOKS

Strengthen your immunity, detox, energize, heal, and stimulate your metabolism with these magical potent healthy recipes!

Get your FREE copy of
"10 Powerful Immune Boosting Recipes"
"12 Healthy Dessert Recipes"
"15 Delicious & Healthy Smoothies"
"The Complete Ayurveda Detox"

Go to *www.MindBodyAndSpiritWellbeing.com* and claim your book!

Or simply scan the QR code below:

Contents

Introduction

We, human beings are very powerful creatures! Our bodies are highly evolved and capable of surviving in different conditions. When one is healthy and energetic, they can achieve anything. But what happens without that life force? What happens when we constantly feel exhausted, sluggish and heavy? Yes, I am talking about chronic fatigue. It has become viral these days. And one of the main reasons is the large quantities of toxins in our bodies.

Today's life is very dynamic and technological. We industrialize, urbanize, utilize, etc. But in our efforts to make everything more efficient, convenient and fast, we have forgotten our roots – nature. Our foods become more genetically and chemically enhanced; the air we breathe is full of only God knows what... Stress, the polluted environment, unhealthy eating habits, medications contaminate our organism. The results are headaches, allergies, joint and back pain, low vitality and poor overall performance. The prognosis for the upcoming decades regarding diseases like cancer, diabetes, cardiovascular conditions, arthritis, infertility, allergies, and so on, are extremely discouraging. My intention here is not to scare anyone. As I already said, our bodies are very powerful! But they are certainly not able to deal with everything. So, in order for them to be healthy, vibrant and strong again, they need a bit of assistance on our side. Fortunately, there is a simple, effective, and easy achievable method to reach this goal. It's called detoxification. There is no coincidence that even spiritual and religious texts advise us to cleanse our bodies at least twice a year! This book is my attempt to help people incorporate different ways of cleansing their precious bodies, so they can have more productive, healthy and fulfilling lives. And more specifically – to do this in small bite-size ways, which can be ingrained in our busy lifestyles.

Which are the most common toxins nowadays?

*M*any substances around us can be considered toxic to our bodies. But we are so used to them, that we cannot really see and feel the difference. We feel tired and reach for the next energy drink that can patch things up. But things do not get any better. For example: I know people who have many cups of strong Italian espresso every day and constantly complain they are sleepy all the time. Their heartbeat accelerates, but they don't have more energy. They wake up tired and irritated, but at night they can't seem to fall asleep easily.

So, here I will name some of the main common toxins, which slow our bodies down. Are you ready?

- Artificial preservatives;
- Artificial colorings;
- Alcohol;
- Drugs and pharmaceuticals – *please consult with your physician before quitting or lowering the dosages of your prescription medications*;
- Cigarettes, cigars, tobacco;
- Caffeine
- Refined sugar;
- White flour and all products from it;
- GMO foods;
- Highly processed foods;
- Artificial sweeteners;
- Air and water pollution;

- Artificial food additives – yes, the vitamins from the pharmacy, too;
- Pesticides, herbicides, and fungicides;
- Meat coming from animals treated with antibiotics and hormones;
- Chemicals in cosmetic products;
- Heavy metals;
- And so on and so on...

I will not describe in detail how these substances affect our bodies. I think we are flooded with information like that. You open the web, or switch on the TV and news like *"Look at this cancerogenic food!"*, *"This drink is poisonous!"*, etc. start to flow. While it is good to be informed, but to my mind, devouring too much negative and scary information can cause more harm (stress), than good. Not to mention how easily we can autosuggest, or become paranoid, or even hypochondriacs. I want to focus on the solutions, which are achievable and give us positive results.

How does the detox work?

*H*ere I will describe very briefly how we naturally cleanse ourselves, so that we can learn how to stimulate and assist this process. Our bodies, as I already mentioned, are very complex and smart organisms. They have developed a perfect mechanism for dealing with harmful external agents. And this responsible task is delegated to the lymphatic system. The job of the lymphatic system is very important – it's the ultimate filter for viruses, bacteria, and fungi. But if we don't cleanse this filter regularly, it becomes congested. This system comprises of multiple tiny vessels, which go in parallel with the blood vessels. It also has a lot of nodes, where multiple lymph vessels join. With this mechanism, the system carries oxygen and nutrients to the cells and takes out all excess fluids. It guards our bodies from malevolent bacteria and viruses. In other words, the lymphatic system has two main jobs. On one hand, it supplies our tissues with precious nutrients, and on the other – flushes out dead cells and harmful agents. It is like the sewer system of the body. This is one of the main reasons why drinking enough water daily is a must for a healthy and cleansed body.

How to decrease the toxin intake?

*R*ealistically speaking at this point of our lifestyles and the state of our environment, completely eliminating toxins from our bodies could be impossible. But it is not even necessary. As I already mentioned, our physical selves are very strong and powerful, beyond what we expect. So, even small changes in our lifestyles can have a profound effect on our health and vitality. We can incrementally start to incorporate some habits, which will decrease the amount of toxic substances we intake. Start applying whatever feels easier to you and build on it as you go. Try to stick with a new habit for at least 30 days, so that you can get used to it.

Here are some examples and ideas:

1. Swap refined sugar with healthier substitutes

The problem with white sugar is not just the calories in it. The main issue comes from the fact that every beneficial ingredient in it has been stripped off – vitamins, microelements, enzymes, etc. This means that our bodies cannot benefit fully from it, moreover, by the process of reverse osmosis, white sugar takes away important substances from our cells. Not to mention the constant insulin rush and its consequences. And since I want to make your life and the detoxing process easier, here I will list some possible sugar substitutes:

a. Fresh or dried fruits – obviously that's the most natural option. Fruits are full of vitamins, microelements, carbohydrates, but also lots of fiber. And fiber is very important. Even though we don't ingest the water insoluble fibers (unlike ruminants), it is still essential for our health and wellbeing. They slow down the absorptions of the carbohydrates and prevent form high blood sugar spikes. They also mechanically, but gently at the same time, brush and stimulate the intestines' walls. This is the main reason why it is best to eat the whole fruits, or drink smoothies, instead of juicing them. Juicing is essential for our detoxing, but it should be a temporary procedure. On a regular day-to-day basis it best for you to ingest the fruits with the fiber (the pulp and the skin). *A word of precaution: some fruits could be very sweet and could raise the blood sugar level even when you ingest the whole fruit. So, if you are diabetic or prone to this disease, try to avoid the sweet sorts of grapes, medlars, dates, pears, bananas, dried figs, raisins, plums, etc. Consult with your dietician or physician for the full list of unsuitable foods for your case.* Speaking of dried fruits, they are excellent for the winter season, but keep in mind they are a highly concentrated food. Also pay attention to the method, in which they were dried, and check if they have any added sugar or preservatives. You can soak them in some warm water for several minutes for them to become juicier. Or if you eat them dry, you will let them absorb the excess water from the body (most dried fruits will bulk and stimulate the intestines, which is a natural and gentle laxative).

b. *Raw honey* – what do I mean by raw honey? It is pure, unprocessed, and unpasteurized honey, straight from the bees' "production line". It contains the most of its nutritious and healing compounds – glucoses, fructose, wide range of vitamins, and loads of minerals (niacin, riboflavin, pantothenic acid, Calcium, Potassium, Copper, Iron, Magnesium, Phosphorus, and Zinc). Different kinds of honey (depending on the plants, from which the bees gathered the pollen) have different healing properties. But all they have in common is that honey is one of the most popular superfood. And it does not spoil! Honey fights the high acidity in the stomach and may heal issues like gastritis and ulcers. It is an antiseptic – it fights infections, bacteria, and fungi. It also strengthens the immune system. There are a few things to be careful with – do not heat honey above the body temperature – it will destroy most of its vitamins and important elements. Also some people may have an allergy to api products (honey, bee pollen, propolis, Gelee Royale, etc.). To prevent this, or to lower the chance of this intolerance, seek honey products, which are pure, coming from clean environment, and without any impurities (some producers mix the honey with other low quality and unwanted compounds, such as potato/corn mash or flour). These extra substances may be the real cause of the allergy, so find a trusted source and test the product with small quantities first. Another thing to consider is the glycemic index

– honey should be taken in small dosages or completely avoided from people with high blood sugar levels.

c. *Maple syrup* - pure Maple syrup is an excellent white sugar substitute. It contains even more minerals than honey (again the essential Calcium, Iron, Manganese, Zinc, Magnesium, Sodium, Potassium, etc.). Actually, there are different types of Maple syrup, divided into grades, depending on the production process and quality. Grade A is the first most natural type, which is the richest in vitamins and minerals. Grade C is more processed, sweeter, and darker. From all natural sugar substitutes, this syrup from the Maple tree is one of the best choices for cooking, because the heat treatment does not affect its quality and beneficial nutrients much. For the purpose of cleansing the body, this natural product is perfect, because it has distinct detoxing properties. It has been used for various natural weight loss and cleansing regimes. It gently assists with the detoxing of the liver, gallbladder, and the kidneys without any side effects. If you retain too much liquid in your body, or suffer from some types of cardio-vascular issues, Maple syrup may help you with its light diuretic effect. Its natural carbohydrates calm the nervous system and balance the hormones. The thing to remember with this product is its high glycemic index – do not use in large quantities. In the next book of the series (Complete Body Cleansing), you can find the annual cleansing program with Maple syrup.

d. Molasses – it is made from sugar beet and sugar cane and it is considered to be a byproduct of the sugar production process. But actually, it turns out molasses contains lots of vitamins and minerals. There are mainly three types of molasses – light, medium dark, and dark, depending on the stage of the production. In the health and bio stores you can find mostly the dark one – it contains less sugar, it has a lower glycemic index, and more minerals and vitamins than the others. On the other hand, it could have a slight bitter taste, so make sure you dilute it in some water. Molasses is suitable for cooking.

e. Brown sugar – it comes from the same sources as white sugar, but there is a main difference – brown sugar is not so highly processed. This means it still contains most of its vitamins, minerals, and enzymes. For example, brown sugar can supply us with Phosphorus, Calcium, Potassium, Iron, Sodium, etc. The things to remember with this white sugar substitute are: it is still sugar and it is not very suitable for people with high blood sugar levels; there are many fake products on the market, which are basically dyed white sugar. Buy from trusted sources and take a good look at its texture – it is usually very sticky (like wet) and stays in large lumps.

f. Coconut sugar – it is produced by the nectar of the coconut palm blossoms. The good news here is that it has relatively low glycemic index. It does not cause such big insulin spikes like other sugary products. It also cannot be processed – coconut sugar is produced by drying the nectar, which naturally crystalizes. This product is full of nutrients, amino acids, Phosphorus, Potassium, Magnesium, Manganese, Copper, and many more beneficial goodies.

g. *Stevia* – this is one of the best natural substitutes for white sugar – it has 0 calories and 0 glycemic index. It is also much sweeter than sugar. You can find it in various forms – liquid, Stevia leaves, tablets, and powder. Choose the one you prefer from trusted sources. This sweet plant is also suitable for cooking and thermal treatment. The even better part of Stevia is its healing properties – it lowers the blood sugar, it is antibacterial and antifungal (excellent for the oral health), strengthens the blood vessels and lowers the blood pressure in the long run, and lowers the chances of osteoporosis development. It is also packed with vitamins and microelements.

h. *Xylitol* – this sugar substitute is quite popular nowadays. I am going to mention it here, but be aware that it has both pros and cons. The main pros of using xylitol are: this natural extract prevents from cavities and mineralizes the teeth; prevents from osteoporosis; its antibacterial properties fight ear infections; it acts as a probiotic – stimulates the growth of beneficial colon bacteria; it is absorbed more slowly than sugar and does not raise the blood sugar level, which makes it perfect for diabetics. Xylitol is a substance found in some fruits and grains, but we don't ingest it in its natural form. It needs to go through various processing for it to become this sugar substitute. This is one of the main reasons many specialists do not accept it as a natural sweetener. And since we cannot absorb it fully, it may cause many abdominal problems and discomforts – cramps, flatulence, even diarrhea. If you choose to use this sugar substitute, try to keep it in small dosages.

i. Agave syrup – this natural sweetener also gains lots of popularity, but it may be considered a bit controversial as well. It is made from a cactus plant. The syrup is sweeter than table sugar, but its glycemic index is lower. It contains lots of minerals and vitamins, which we can absorb fully – vitamins K, A, B, D, E; essential elements like Iron, Magnesium, Calcium, Potassium, Phosphorus, Sodium, Zinc, Copper, Selenium, etc. This sugar substitute also stimulates the bowel movement, soothes neuralgias, takes out excess water from the body, and assists the respiratory and digestive tracts. The important things to remember about this sweet syrup are: read the labels carefully – most of the Agave syrups on the market contain a lot of fructose and are highly processed (like white sugar). Choose the ones, which are raw and had not been processed with high temperatures. Logically raw Agave syrup is not suitable for cooking, because it will destroy most of its beneficial substances and it will transform into glucoses.

Some white sugar substitutes to stay away from – Aspartame, Fructose (glucose-fructose syrup, or corn syrup), Acesulfame K, Cyclamate, Sucralose, Sorbitol (E420), Maltilol (E965), Erythritol (should not be used frequently and in large quantities),

Brown rice syrup (although it contains some minerals, its glycemic index is high, and it's highly processed; if you decide to use it, do it in moderation).

Also, do yourself and your body a huge favor and start switching from sodas and juices to water and herbal teas. Bonus! You will even save some money!

If you need some ideas to include the healthier white sugar alternatives in your diet, take a look at these suggestions:

Dry Fruits Candy

Ingredients:
1 1/2 cup **dry fruits** of choice (apricots, plums, raisins, etc.)
6 1/2 Tbsps. **grated walnuts**
3 Tbsps. **desiccated coconut** or sesame seeds
2 Tbsps. **cocoa powder**
3 Tbsps. **butter**
4 1/2 Tbsps. grade B **maple syrup**
1/2 cup **oat meal**
1 cup **dry milk**
2 cups **warm water**

Instructions:
Choose dry fruits without any additional sugar or fructose syrup. Wash them carefully and soak them in some boiling water for 20 minutes. After that wash them again with cold water, and grind them in

a food processor or a blender. Mix the cocoa powder, the maple syrup, dry milk, and the oat meal and stir well. Add the warm water and blend the ingredients. Place the mixture in a double boiler and stir well until it becomes completely homogenous. Next add the butter, the fruits, and stir again. Take the mixture off the heat and let it cool off. Form small candy balls and dip them in the desiccated coconut, sesame, and/or walnuts.

Nutty Candy Balls

Ingredients:
1 cup **raisins**
1 cup **walnuts**
1 bio **organic orange**
2 Tbsps. **honey**
Some **sesame seeds,** desiccated coconut, or cocoa powder

Instructions:
Grind the nuts and place them in a big bowl. Peel the orange and grind its zest. Place the raisins in a blender or kitchen chopper and mince them. Next, add the orange zest and the honey to the raisins and blend them. Take the mixture and combine it with the walnuts in the bowl. Stir well and blend the ingredients. With moist hands form balls from the nutty "dough" and cover them with the sesame seeds, desiccated coconut, or cocoa powder. Place the nutty candies in the fridge for 2-3 hours.

Energy Bars with Walnut Tahini

Ingredients:
1 1/2 cup **walnut tahini** (or ground raw walnuts)
1 cup **sunflower seeds** (or sunflower tahini)
1/2 cup **honey**, maple or agave syrup
3 Tbsps. **carob powder**
6 Tbsps. **coconut butter** (melted)
A pinch of **Himalayan salt**

Instructions:
Mix all ingredients in a blender or kitchen chopper and mince them well. Take the "dough" and form it in the desired shapes. Place them in the fridge for a couple of hours.

Extra Strong Energy Balls with Chestnuts

Ingredients:
2 cups **chestnuts**
1 **coconut**
20 **dates**
1 Tbsp. **honey**
3-4 Tbsps. **Sesame seeds**
2-3 Tbsps. **Flax seeds**
1-2 Tbsps. **Chia seeds**
3-4 Tbsps. **Poppy seeds**
1/2 cup **water**
Some **cocoa powder**

Instructions:

First, boil and peel the chestnuts. Depending on the chestnuts, they may need from 15 to 35 minutes to be completely cooked.

Next, grind the seeds – the flax, sesame, and chia seeds.

Now take the "meat" from the coconut and mince it in a kitchen chopper.

Next, mix the seeds powder, the chestnuts, and the coconut in a large bowl, and blend them with a hand mixer. Add some water to make the process easier.

Remove the pits of the dates and add the fruits to the mix along with the honey. Continue to stir with the mixer.

Finally, add the poppy seeds and stir with a spoon.

Place the bowl in the fridge for about half an hour to harden a little bit.

Start forming small balls with the desired size and volume. Dip and roll them in the cocoa powder to be fully covered. Bring the candies back in the fridge to keep their proper shape.

My notes:

Yummy Lenten Apple Cake

Ingredients:
1 cup **raw walnuts**
4 Tbsps. **Honey** or agave syrup
1 Tbsp. **cinnamon**
4 **apples**
4 Tbsps. **raw cashews**

Instructions:

Grind the walnuts and mix them with the honey and half of the cinnamon powder. You will reach a sticky pliable "dough" consistency. Spread the cake crust at about 2 cm (3/4 inch) thick in a baking pan.

Grate the apples and mix them with the remaining cinnamon. Put the apple mixture on top of the crust.

Grind the cashews and sprinkle them on top of the cake.

My notes:

Fiber Candy with Flax Seeds

Ingredients:
1 cup **oat meal**
1 cup **desiccated coconut**
1/2 cup bio **dark chocolate chips**
1/2 cup **peanut butter**
1/2 cup **flax seeds**, ground or crushed
1/3 cup **honey**
1 tsp. **vanilla extract**

Instructions:
Simply mix all ingredients in a large bowl. Stir and knead them well until the "dough" becomes fully homogenous. Place the mixture in the fridge for half an hour. Next, take the mix out and form small candy balls or other forms, and enjoy!
Store the candy in the fridge!

My notes:

Chickpeas Candy

Ingredients:
1/2 cup **dry plums**
5 drops liquid **vanilla extract**
1/2 cup **boiled chickpeas**
1/2 cup **sesame seeds**
6 Tbsps. **cocoa powder**
1/4 cup **honey**
A pinch of ground sea or Himalayan **salt**

Instructions:
Mix the boiled chickpeas (they should not be hot), the plums, the cocoa, and the honey in a blender or food processor. Add the vanilla, the salt, and blend the ingredients until the mixture becomes smooth. Form small balls (or any other desired shapes), cover them with sesame seeds, and place them in the fridge. In a couple of hours the candies are ready for consumption.

My notes:

Chocolate Truffles

Ingredients:
1 cup **buckwheat flour**
1 cup **yogurt**
1/2 cup **dry plums** (without the kernels)
1 Tbsp. **brown/coconut sugar**, honey, or maple syrup
2 Tbsps. **cocoa powder**
1 tsp. **sunflower oil**
1/2 tsp. **baking soda**
1 1/2 tsps. **vanilla sugar**
Some **sesame seeds**

Instructions:
Pour some hot water on the dry plums, let them soak for about half an hour, and puree them with a hand blender. Add the yogurt and the sunflower oil. In a large bowl mix the buckwheat flour, baking soda, the sugar, the cocoa, and the vanilla sugar. Add the liquid puree (from the plums and yogurt) to the mix and stir well. You will need to reach a thick dough consistency. Form small candy balls (or other shapes). Cover the candies with sesame seeds and place them in a baking pan with oiled paper. Bake the cookies for 15 minutes in a preheated oven (at 180 deg. C/ 356 F). Voila!

Pumpkin Truffles

Ingredients:
1 cup **boiled pumpkin**
1 cup **ground almonds**
1 cup **ground walnuts**
1 Tbsp. **sesame tahini**
2 Tbsps. **honey**
1 tsp. **cinnamon**
3 Tbsps. **Desiccated coconut**
1 Tbsp. **cocoa powder**
1 Tbsp. **melted coconut butter**
More **cocoa powder** and **desiccated coconut** for the coating

Instructions:
Simply mix all ingredients in a large bowl and blend them well. If the mixture is too runny, you can add more nuts and tahini. Shape small balls and cover them with the cocoa powder or the desiccated coconut.

Place them in the fridge for at least 1 hour to keep their shape.

My notes:

Oat Meal Candy Bars

Ingredients:
2 cups **oat meal**
1/2 cup **dry plums** (without the kernels)
1/2 cup **raw walnuts**
Some **hot pure water**
Some **coconut sugar** or maple syrup according to your taste

Instructions:
Note: choose dry plums without any sugar, artificial sweeteners or other chemicals.

Cut the plums in small pieces and grind the walnuts. Mix the oat meal, the plums, and the walnuts in a bowl. Mix the hot water and the natural sweetener. Stir until the sugar/maple syrup is fully melted. Slowly add the sweet water until you reach a thick paste. Place the "dough" in a well-oiled pan. Place the pan on the stove on very low heat. Cover the pan with a lid and let the paste cook on both sides for 7-10 minutes. Be careful not to burn it. When you reach a nice golden crust, the dessert is ready. Take it off the heat, wait for it to cool off, and cut it in pieces.

Chocolate Candy with Milk Cream

Ingredients:
2 cups **coconut sugar** or maple syrup
1 cup **dry milk**
4 Tbsps. **butter**
1 tsp. **vanilla**
Bio **dark chocolate**

Instructions:
Mix all ingredients in a pot (without the chocolate) and melt them on low heat. Stir well until everything is fully blended. Form small candies in the desired form and put them in a baking pan covered with oiled paper. Bake the cookies at 180 deg. C (356 F) for 10-15 minutes. The oven has to be preheated and keep an eye on the candies. They can burn easily. Take the candies out of the oven and let them cool off. In the meantime, melt the chocolate and cover the candies with it. Place the desserts in the fridge to harden the icing.

My notes:

Healthy Raw Chocolate 1

Ingredients:
1/2 cup **raw cacao paste**
2 cups **raw cocoa butter**
1/4 cup **agave syrup**
1 tsp. **Maca powder**
2 tsps. **Coconut butter**
1/2 cup **raw cashew**

Instructions:
Grate the cacao paste and the cocoa butter. Place them in a double boiler and melt them. Be careful not to let the water boil and burn the ingredients. Next, finely grind the cashew and add it to the cocoa mix. Add all remaining ingredients and stir well. When everything is fully blended, pour the mixture into suitable molds and let the chocolate cool off.

My notes:

Healthy Raw Chocolate 2 (with Superfoods)

Ingredients:
5 Tbsps. **raw cacao paste**
4 tsps. **raw cocoa butter**
8 tsps. **honey**
2 Tbsps. **Raw almonds**
2 Tbsps. **Goji berries**
1 tsp. grated **lemon zest**

Instructions:
Grind the almonds. If you wish, you can grind the berries as well. Next, place the cacao paste and the cocoa butter in a double boiler and let them melt completely. Take the mixture off the heat and add the honey, the almonds, the Goji berries and the lemon zest. Stir well to blend all ingredients. Pour the chocolate in suitable molds and place it in the fridge until it hardens.

My notes:

Cocoa Mixture

Ingredients:
2 cups **raw sunflower seeds**
1/2 cup **raw almonds**
1 cup **raisins**
2 Tbsps. **Flax seeds**
2 Tbsps. **Coconut butter**
1 inch **ginger root**
2 Tbsps. **Cocoa powder**
1 Tbsp. **cinnamon**
water

Instructions:
Take the seeds and nuts (sunflower, flax, almonds, and raisins) and soak them in pure water for several hours. Then, wash them thoroughly and mince them in a kitchen chopper.

Peel the ginger root and cut it in pieces. Add it in the chopper (or blender) along with all remaining ingredients. Add some water to reach the desired consistency. Blend everything well until it is fully homogenous.

My notes:

Dairy Dessert with Curd

Ingredients:
1 1/2 cup **dry curd**

1/2 cup **dark bio chocolate** (without white sugar)

1 cup **liquid cream**

2 Tbsps. **soft butter**

1/2 cup **coconut sugar** or maple syrup

Instructions:

If you are using coconut sugar, grind it in a coffee grinder or a kitchen chopper to reach a powdered consistency. Mix the curd, the butter, the sugar, and the cream in a bowl and blend them well. Use a blender if necessary. The end result needs to be dry without any dripping liquids. If the curd is not dry enough, add more cream and butter. Use the mixture to form any desired shapes and place the candies in the freezer for 20 minutes.

In the meantime, we will prepare the icing. Melt the chocolate in a double boiler on low heat. Add some liquid cream and stir well. Next, take it off the heat and let it cool off a little bit. Take out the candies, dip them in the melted chocolate and bring them back in the freezer. Let their icing harden there for an hour, and then, move the desserts to the fridge.

Dairy Candies

Ingredients:
1 1/2 cup **dry milk**

2 Tbsps. **cocoa powder**

2 Tbsps. **soft butter**

3 Tbsps. cow or vegetable **milk**

1 1/2 cup **ground nuts** of choice – walnuts, almonds, cashew, etc.

1 cup **maple syrup** or coconut sugar

Instructions:
Mix the liquid milk, the maple syrup/sugar, and the cocoa powder in a metal pot and heat it. Stir continuously until the mixture starts to simmer. Next, take it off the heat and add the nuts, and the butter. Stir and slowly add the dry milk while mixing. The goal is to reach a dough-like consistency. Start kneading the mixture until everything is fully blended. Take a clean plate and cover it with wrapping kitchen foil and sprinkle some dry milk on top. Start forming small candy balls from the "dough" and put them in the plate. Cover the desserts with foil and place the dish in the fridge for 1-2 hours.

My notes:

Sesame Dairy Bars

Ingredients:
1/2 cup **sesame seeds**
1 cup **butter**
1/2 cup **dry milk**
5 Tbsps. **coconut sugar/maple syrup**

Instructions:
Note: if you are using coconut sugar, grind it beforehand to reach a powder consistency.

Place the butter in a pan, melt it, and let it simmer on low heat. Do not forget to stir to avoid burning the grease. Now add the sesame seeds while you keep stirring. When the seeds start to become golden brown, add the dry milk and the sugar. Stir again to fully blend all ingredients.

Next, pour the mixture in an oiled baking pan or a plate, and place it in the fridge. In 30 minutes, you can take it out of the fridge and cut it in the desired shapes.

My notes:

Raw Cinnamon Rolls

Ingredients:
1 cup **raw walnuts**
4 Tbsps. **honey**
1 Tbsp. **cinnamon**
4 **apples**
4 Tbsps. **raw almonds**

Instructions:
Mix the walnuts, the honey, and half of the cinnamon in a kitchen chopper and blend them. The result will be a sticky pliable mixture. Spread the "dough" in a baking form.

Next, grate the apples and mix them with the remaining cinnamon. Spread evenly the mixture on top of the walnut "dough". Now grind the almonds and sprinkle them on top of the apple layer. Gently roll the layers and form a nice sweet cinnamon roll. Place it in the fridge to harden a little bit. Cut it in several pieces and enjoy!

My notes:

----

2. Start including more fresh fruits and vegetables in your diet

Eliminating highly processed foods is a big step towards more energy and better health. Unfortunately, they are so addictive! It has been scientifically proven that our brain treats sugar, fried food, trans fats, and artificial preservatives, coloring etc. the same way it treats drugs! Now that explains a lot! This does not mean we should give up the battle and make just another excuse! *"It's not my fault! It's an addiction! I can't help but eat... this and that..."* We have the capacity to overcome any vice! Be smart and try different approaches. Rash changes are stressful for the body, so try with small steps. For example, have one salad a day for at least 30 consecutive days. Think about healthier alternatives to your favorite foods and start swapping. Another example: whenever you feel a craving for some junk food, eat something healthy first. Later on, the body will make the connection, and before you know it, your receptors will have changed and your cravings will be rarer and rarer. In my next detox book you will find more information about which foods have the best cleansing properties. But for now, for the purpose of beginning a healthier lifestyle, more fresh fruits and vegetables is quite enough.

The best and easiest way to include more fruits and veggies in our diets is smoothies. They are delicious, healthy, refreshing, and full of vitamins, minerals, and enzymes. Here are some sample recipes you can try:

Green Smoothie with Basil

Ingredients:
1 big **ripe avocado**
Some **fresh basil leaves**
1 cup **almond milk**
2 **lemons**
1 Tbsp. **honey**
Some **crushed ice cubes** (optional)

Instructions:
Cut the avocado in medium cubes and squeeze the juice from the lemons. Place the avocado, the lemon juice, the basil, almond milk, and the honey in a blender and stir until the mixture is fully homogenous. The smoothie is ready! You can add the ice cubes to make the healthy beverage even more refreshing during the hot season!

Green Smoothie with Einkorn bran

Ingredients:
2 1/2 cups **bio yogurt** (preferably Bulgarian or Greek)
1 cup **low fat curd**
2 ripe **bananas**
1 cup **spinach**
3 Tbsps. **einkorn bran**
3 Tbsps. **honey**

Instructions:
Wash the spinach thoroughly and remove the stems. We will be using only the leaves. Place the spinach, the yogurt, bananas (cut in pieces), and the curd in a blender and stir. Next, add the einkorn bran and the honey, and mix again until everything is fully blended.

Green Smoothie with Avocado

Ingredients:
1 **ripe avocado**
1 cup **pineapple**
1 cup **fresh spinach**
1 **banana**
1/2 cup **almond milk**

Instructions:
Peel and cut the fruits in pieces. Wash the spinach thoroughly with clean water. Place all ingredients in a blender and stir.

My notes:

Stinging Nettle Smoothie

Ingredients:
A fistful of **fresh young Stinging nettle leaves**
A fistful of **fresh parsley**
1 **banana**
1 **apple**
1 **orange**
1 cup **pure water**
Some **seeds** – sesame, flax seeds, poppy, etc.

Instructions:
Peel the fruits (you can skip the apple), and cut them in pieces. Place them in a blender. Wash the leafy greens carefully and add them in the blender. Add the water and stir until you reach a smooth consistency. Pour in glasses and garnish with the desired seeds.

This smoothie is extremely healthy and refreshing, with acute anti-aging and weight-loss properties.

My notes:

Spinach Smoothie with Pineapple

Ingredients:
1/2 cup **fresh pineapple**
1 cup **coconut milk**
2 Tbsps. **Desiccated coconut**
1 cup **spinach**
1 Tbsp. **Flax seeds**

Instructions:
Grind the flax seeds. Peel and cut the pineapple in pieces. Now mix all ingredients in a blender and stir. Pour in suitable glasses and decorate with some desiccated coconut.

Nutty Smoothie with Spinach

Ingredients:
1 cup **yogurt** (preferably Bulgarian)
1/2 **banana**
1/2 **apple**
1/4 cup (a fistful) **spinach**
1 Tbsp. **walnuts, almonds, cedar, or other nuts**
1/2 cup **water**

Instructions:
Peel the banana and cut it with the apple in large pieces. Place the fruits in a blender, add the yogurt, the spinach, and mince them well. Add some water to reach the desired consistency and blend

again. Garnish the smoothie with the chosen nuts (grind them beforehand).

Veggie Smoothie

Ingredients:
1/2 head of **lettuce**
3 **tomatoes**
5 cm (2 inch) **cucumber**
1/2 **lemon**
A fistful of **parsley**

Instructions:
Peel the lemon, cut it in pieces and remove any seeds. Wash all vegetables and cut them in pieces. Place all ingredients in the blender and stir well until everything is fully homogenous.

Pineapple & Walnuts Smoothie

Ingredients:
1/2 **medium pineapple**
1 **apple** (preferably green)
1 **banana**
1 cup **water**
1 Tbsp. **fresh lemon juice**
Some **raw walnuts** according to your taste

Instructions:

Peel and cut the fruits (you can leave the apple's skin). Place all ingredients in a blender and stir until you reach a smooth consistency. The quantities will yield about 4 cups of smoothie. Store the remaining liquid in the fridge and consume until the end of the day.

Sweet Carrot Smoothie 1

Ingredients:
A fistful of **raw walnuts**
2 **average carrots**
1 **banana**
1/4 **pineapple**
Some **soy or almond milk**

Instructions:
Peel the carrots and fruits, and cut them in pieces. Place all ingredients in a blender and stir.

My notes:

Sweet Carrot Smoothie 2

Ingredients:
1/4 cup **apple juice**
1 cup **carrot juice**
1 **banana**
1 cup **yogurt or kefir**
Some **cinnamon or vanilla**

Instructions:
Mix all ingredients in a blender and stir well. When the mixture becomes smooth and homogenous, the healthy drink is ready!

Pumpkin Smoothie 1

Ingredients:
1 **banana**
1 **carrot**
1-2 stalks **celery** (with the leaves)
A piece of **fresh pumpkin**
1/2 tsp. **cinnamon**
1 cup **water**

Instructions:
Wash and peel the fruits and veggies carefully. Cut them in pieces and put them in a blender. Add the water and the cinnamon and stir well.

Note: fresh pumpkin can be a little bit harsh on the stomach and the gastrointestinal tract. If you have any health issues in this area, bake the pumpkin beforehand and consult with your physician!

Pumpkin Smoothie 2

Ingredients:
1 cup **pumpkin puree**
1 1/2 cup cow/goat or vegetable **milk**
2 **bananas**
1 Tbsp. **ground flax seeds**
1/4 cup **oat meal**
1 tsp. **cinnamon**
1/4 tsp. **nutmeg powder**
Some **honey** (optional)

Instructions:
Peel the bananas and cut them in pieces. Put them in a blender; add the flax seeds, and the oat meal. Pour the milk and add the spices. Stir well until everything is fully blended. Serve and consume right away.

Note: fresh pumpkin can be a little bit harsh on the stomach and the gastrointestinal tract. If you have any health issue in this area, bake the pumpkin beforehand and consult with your physician!

Apple & Oats Smoothie

Ingredients:
1 cup **fresh apple juice**
1 **banana**
3 Tbsps. **oat meal**
Some **pumpkin or sunflower seeds**

Instructions:
Peel the banana and cut it in pieces. Place all ingredients in a blender and stir well.

Persimmon Yogurt Shake 1

Ingredients:
2 cups **persimmons**
1 1/2 cup **yogurt**
1 **banana**
1 Tbsp. **oat meal**

Instructions:
Cut the persimmons and remove any seeds. Peel the banana and cut it in pieces. Place the fruits, the yogurt and the oat meal in a blender and stir. When the mixture becomes homogenous, the shake is ready.

Persimmon Yogurt Shake 2

Ingredients:
2 average **persimmons**
8 Tbsps. **yogurt**
2 average **bananas**
1 **orange**

Instructions:
Squeeze the juice from the orange. Next, peel the fruits and remove any seeds from the persimmons. Cut the fruits in pieces and put them in a blender and stir. Next, add the orange juice and the yogurt. Stir again until you reach a homogenous mixture.

Healthy Aromatic Ayurveda Shake

Ingredients:
1 cup **yogurt**
1/2 cup **water**
1 cup **fresh fruits** of choice
2 Tbsps. **Honey or carob powder**
A pinch of **cardamom**
1/2 tsp. **vanilla extract**
4-5 **saffron stigmas**
1 Tbsp. **almond milk**
A pinch of **grated lemon zest** (optional)

Instructions:

First we need to dilute the saffron – it requires some time to develop its taste and health properties. Place it in the almond milk the night before.

The next day, place all ingredients in a blender and mince them well.

Pour in glasses and enjoy!

Coconut Smoothie with Chicory Coffee

Ingredients:

4-5 Tbsps. **Chicory coffee**
1 **banana**
2-3 Tbsps. **Coconut milk**
1 1/2 Tbsps. **Desiccated coconut**
1 tsp. **honey**

Instructions:

Peel the banana and cut it in pieces. Place all ingredients in a blender and stir.

Note: the coffee needs to be at room temperature, so it won't destroy the healthy nutrients in the honey.

My notes:

----

3. Don't keep junk food at home/office

Just think about where you spend most of your time and keep this space junk food free. This will lower the chances of having unhealthy meals. Because let's face it – we humans are a bit lazy – if something is easily available, quick, and in a short distance, we will choose that instead of something, which takes time and effort to make. If we stash unhealthy foods, ready for munching, the temptation is almost irresistible. But if we store only what is good for us, it is much easier to keep a healthier lifestyle, especially when we have cravings. The same principle applies for our workspace. If we don't have easy access to healthy options, we usually choose the junk food. That is why fast food restaurants do so well these days. But don't worry, you can make your own healthy fast food. For example, fruits, nuts, seeds, salads (previously cut), or something prepared at home, suitable for your work environment. There are tons of recipes, books, and ideas on the matter. When I applied this principle at home, I found a great change in my eating habits. I stopped keeping sugar and other unhealthy foods at home. And when I have a sweet craving, I take scoop from my honey jar and combine it with some sunflower/pumpkin seed/sesame tahini, or even better – I eat some fruits. Now I don't crave sugar as much I did before.

4. Substitute white flour with healthier options

The problem with white flour is very similar to the one with white sugar – it is low on beneficial nutrients, minerals, enzymes, and has no fiber, which causes blood sugar spikes. Not to mention how genetically modified the wheat grains are. Another sad tendency is the increasing amount of people who experience gluten intolerance. One way or another, these people should look for more suitable alternatives. The good news is that nowadays more and more stores and bakeries supply healthy GMO-free products, raw bars, etc. The market is full of whole grain bread and pasta! Start making different choices! To tell you the truth, whole grain bread tastes much better than the common white bread! If you can go without any pastries, even better! You won't notice how and where these extra pounds went! If you ran out of ideas, here I will list some suggestions for healthier white flour substitutes:

a. *Einkorn and Emmer* – these are actually types of wheat, but they are very different from what we eat today. These are old sorts of cereals, which are very close to the natural wild ones. They are the first cultivated types of wheat, which makes them GMO-free. And we all know what GMO foods do our bodies. I also feel there is a direct connection between GMO wheat products and gluten intolerance. For example – soy (which now is highly genetically modified) – researches show that soy consumption causes a 50% spike of allergies for peanuts (soy and peanuts are like cousins).

b. *Buckwheat flour* – if you have never tried buckwheat, and you want to live a healthier life, I advise you to pay extra attention to this tiny seed. It is packed with beneficial nutrients and has distinct healing properties. It contains around

14% proteins, healthy fats, fiber, vitamins A, B, E, PP, microelements – Iron, Calcium, Phosphorus, Iodine, Boron, Magnesium, and Zinc, and organic acids such as citric and malic, but it does not contain gluten. This natural product is perfect for weight loss for its fiber content. It is also suitable for decreasing the blood sugar and blood pressure levels. Buckwheat is also beneficial for people suffering from anemia, gastritis, flatulence, gallstones, varicose veins, hemorrhoids, constipation, gout, rheumatism, nephritis, etc. It also supports and cleanses the liver and kidneys, regulates the work of the thyroid, helps with the reduction of cellulite, and even prevents from cancer cell formation. Of course every healthy food has its proper dosages. Be careful with consuming Buckwheat if you have ulcers (stomach or duodenal), or if you are pregnant or breastfeeding. Large quantities of this plant can provoke photosensitivity.

c. *Almond powder* – this one does not contain gluten, it is GMO-free, and it is packed with vitamin E. The downside of it is its short shelf life. You need to store it in a refrigerator, or freeze it after opening the package, if you don't plan to use it any time soon.

d. *Quinoa flour* – now we all know how healthy the quinoa grains are – they contain all essential amino acids, which makes them perfect alternative for vegetarians and vegans. You don't need to abstain from meat, eggs, and dairy products for you to indulge in consuming this gluten-free and GMO-free plant. The thing to consider with quinoa is its slightly bitter taste. To avoid that, bake the powder beforehand on oiled paper for 10 min. at 100 degrees Celsius (212 F).

e. *Hemp flour* – it will take me several pages to describe how beneficial this plant is for us, but I will keep it short. In a few words – hemp seeds are full of amino acids, vitamins, and micro elements – Zinc, Magnesium, Silicon, Chrome, Germanium, Calcium, Iron, and many more. Plus they don't contain gluten and usually are not genetically modified. These precious little grains are excellent food for lowering the blood pressure and blood sugar level, strengthening the immune system, and cleansing the colon (without harming the good bacteria), enhancing the eyesight, and so many other benefits. Two things to remember about hemp seeds. One – keep the doses small and do not use it daily, overdosing may cause diarrhea, and even hemorrhages. Two – hemp seeds are rich in Omega-3 amino acids, this is usually very good, but they act as a natural blood thinner. This should be noted by people who take anticoagulant medications, and they must be very careful with this white flour substitute.

f. *Chestnut powder* – one of the best healthy flour alternatives, which are suitable for people with a gluten allergy. Surprisingly, chestnuts contain as much Vitamin C as lemons. They are also packed with Phosphorus and Potassium, which support the nervous system. Also you can find lots of antioxidants, which fight various diseases and slow down the aging process. Chestnuts are well known in natural medicine – they counteract issues like anemia, and diarrhea.

g. *Chickpeas flour* – this product is not news for human kind. Chickpeas are popular among the eastern nations and Italy. This flour substitute is an excellent choice for healthy pizzas and focaccias. Chickpeas are so nutritious and beneficial for our bodies, I don't know where to begin with their values. First of all, they are rich in fiber, which cleanses the colon, lowers the cholesterol and blood sugar levels, and (of course) promotes weight loss. These small peas are a great asset for vegetarians and vegans for their large quantities of plant proteins. Chickpeas give you energy, because of its Manganese and Iron supplies (excellent for anemic people). Women should really consider using these legumes, because of their antioxidants and many microelements (Iron, Phosphorus, Calcium, Magnesium, Zinc, Vitamin K), which prevent from osteoporosis and female hormone imbalances. There are some researches, which show proofs that chickpeas promote cancer cells' death, support the natural detox processes, and sooth inflammations (because of the containing choline).

h. *Amaranth powder* – Amaranth is very similar to the quinoa grains – it contains lots of proteins, fiber, vitamins, and minerals (Magnesium, Phosphorus, Calcium, Iron, etc.). It is easily digestible, and it's suitable even for children and people with gastro enteric problems. One of its best qualities is the absence of gluten, which makes it perfect for people with such allergy. Amaranth supports and nourishes the body, and it could be a valuable part of the healthy diet for people who do heavy physical or stressful work, or those who exercise regularly.

i. ***Oat meal and oat bran*** – they are commonly known for their health and weight loss benefits. A research published in Molecular Nutrition & Food Research shows that some compounds in oat meal (glucans) lower the appetite by stimulating the hormones, which fight hunger (cholecystokinin). They also assist with counteracting hypertension, by lowering the cholesterol plaques. Oat meal is extremely beneficial for the skin – it contains vitamin K, vitamins from group B, Zinc, and carotene, which make the derma smooth, and promote its regeneration. Its large quantities of fiber cleanse the colon (especially oat bran) and prevent from cancer in this area. It also boosts our energy, strengthens the immune system, and helps us have a restful good night sleep. The only downside of oat meal is the containing gluten. You can choose oat bran, which contains far less gluten, less calories, and much more fiber.

j. ***Teff flour*** – I left this relatively new type of flour for last. It is still not so common, but it has a great potential. Teff could be considered a superfood – it is loaded with beneficial elements like Calcium, and vitamin C. It contains lots of fiber, which regulates the blood sugar and cholesterol levels, and supports and cleanses the colon. Plus it is gluten-free.

Here are some recipes with white flour substitutes you can try:

Banana Pancakes

Ingredients:
3 Tbsps. **corn/oat meal/oat bran powder**
1 **banana**
150 ml (~1/2 cup) **soy milk**
1 **egg**
1 tsp. **baking soda**
1 Tbsp. **coconut butter**

Instructions:
Melt the coconut butter and mix with all other ingredients. Blend them well until the mixture is fully homogenous. Bake the pancakes in a non-stick frying pan, preferably without using any additional fat.

My notes:

Wholegrain Fiber Pancakes

Ingredients:
1/2 cup **wholegrain einkorn/emmer flour**
1/4 cup **oat bran**
1 Tbsp. **ground flax seeds**
1 Tbsp. **baking powder**
1 tsp. **cinnamon/nutmeg**
1 tsp. **vanilla**
1 cup **almond milk**
2-3 Tbsps. grade B **maple syrup**

Instructions:
Mix all dry ingredients in a bowl – the flour, the oat bran, flax seeds, baking powder, cinnamon, and vanilla extract. Mix the maple syrup with the almond milk and stir until the sweetener dissolves. Add the sweet liquid to the dry ingredients and stir well. When you reach a homogenous consistency, you can start baking the pancakes. Use a non-stick pan and avoid using any oils.

My notes:

Wholegrain Diet Pancakes

Ingredients:
4 **eggs**
1 cup **cottage cheese or curd**
2 Tbsps. **Wholegrain flour of choice** – emmer, einkorn, spelt, etc.
Some **butter or ghee** (optional)

Instructions:
Mix all ingredients in a large suitable bowl. Stir well with a mixer until everything is fully blended. Let the mélange sit for at least 5 minutes.

Take a non-stick frying pan and bake the pancakes. You can grease the pan with some butter to make them extra smooth. Remember to turn them very carefully, so that they do not fall apart or burn.

Serve with fruits or some honey, agave/maple syrup, homemade chocolate (see the recipe in the healthy sugar substitutes recipes section).

My notes:

Fast and Easy Cake

Ingredients:
2 cups **wholegrain einkorn/emmer/spelt flour**
2 Tbsps. **ground flax seeds**
4 Tbsps. **raisins**
1/2 cup **raw walnuts**
1 1/2 cup **yogurt**
1 tsp. **baking soda**
A pinch of **nutmeg**
1/2 tsp. **cinnamon**
1 tsp. **grated lemon zest**
5 Tbsps. **Ghee butter**
5 Tbsps. **Carob powder**

Instructions:
Soak the raisins in some water for a couple of hours.

Next, grind the walnuts and mix them with the flour, the flax seeds, the carob powder, the lemon zest, the nutmeg, and the cinnamon in a large bowl.

In another container mix the yogurt and the baking soda. Stir well until the baking soda is fully dissolved. Remember that the container has to be larger than the yogurt, because the mixture will start to rise and froth.

Next, put the yogurt mixture in the bowl with the flour and spices. Mix well the ingredients.

Melt the ghee butter on low temperature. When it's ready, add it to the mixture. Now strain the raisins and add them to the dough as well and stir.

Take a baking form, grease it with some oil or butter, and cover it with some flour. Next, pour the cake mixture inside and bake for about 45-50 minutes at 180 deg. C (356 F).

Homemade Wholegrain Pasta

Ingredients:
1 **egg**
1 cup **wholegrain spelt flour**
2 Tbsps. **wholegrain emmer or einkorn flour**
1/2 tsp. **salt** – ground sea or Himalayan salt
1 Tbsp. **olive oil**

Instructions:
Use a sieve and sift the flours – any large particles will ruin the dough's consistency. Place the flour in a large bowl or directly on the clean kitchen counter. Form a hole and place the egg yolk, egg white, the salt and the olive oil inside. Start mixing the ingredients and knead the dough. It will have a thick consistency. Next, divide the mixture in 4 equal parts, cover them with a towel or stretch foil and let them sit for about half an hour.

Next, take each dough ball, press it gently and run it through a pasta maker. First start with the large grades and then use the smaller ones. In-between each pressing, sprinkle the dough with some flour to avoid it from becoming sticky.

If you do not have a pasta machine, use a rolling pin to reach a thin film of dough.

Cut the pasta in the desired forms and let it dry for at least 20-30 minutes and the pasta is ready for cooking! Boil this Italian deliciousness for 3-4 minutes in boiling water with 2-3 Tbsps. olive oil.

Here are some ideas for your delicious and healthy wholegrain pasta!

Mediterranean Tagliatelle with Shrimps

Ingredients:
400 grams (1 1/2 – 2 cups) **homemade wholegrain pasta**
300 grams (1 – 1 1/2 cups) **shrimps**
2 average **zucchinis**
2 cloves **garlic**
4-5 Tbsps. **olive oil**
80 ml (5 tbsps.) **white wine**
80 ml (5 tbsps.) **pasta bullion** (the water from the boiled pasta)
1 **egg yolk**
Salt and pepper

Instructions:

Boil the pasta in pure water with some salt and 2-3 tbsps. olive oil. Strain it and keep some of the water.

Peel the zucchinis and cut them in thin strips. Put some olive oil in a large frying pan (such as the wok) and heat it. Add the zucchinis and the garlic cloves. In several minutes take them off the heat, remove the veggies with a slotted spoon, and sprinkle them with some salt. Next, put the shrimps in the same frying pan, fry them for 2-3 minutes, add the wine and bring back the zucchinis. Cook them for about a minute more, add some more olive oil, the strained tagliatelle, and 5 tbsps. of the pasta bullion. Stir well and cook the pasta for 1-2 more minutes.

Next, take the dish off the heat, let it cool off for 4-5 minutes and add the egg yolk, the pepper, and stir.

If you like, you can grate some parmesan on top.

My notes:

Baked Macaroni

Ingredients:

1 cup **wholegrain macaroni or homemade pasta**

3 tbsps. **coconut butter**

3 cups **almond milk**

1 tsp. **vanilla extract**

3 **eggs**

6 Tbsps. grade B **maple syrup or coconut sugar**

1 cup **soy tofu** (optional)

Instructions:

Boil the pasta in water with some salt and oil of choice, and strain it. In a bowl mix all remaining ingredients and blend them well. Put the mixture in a baking pan with the macaroni. Bake the pasta in a preheated oven (180 deg. C/356 F) until you have a nice golden crust.

My notes:

Italian Tuna Salad

Ingredients:
2 cups **wholegrain macaroni or homemade pasta**
1 average fresh **red pepper**
1 small **bulb onion**
Some fresh **parsley**
Some ground **Himalayan salt** according to your taste
1/2-1 cup **tuna fillet**
1 1/2 cup **boiled sweet corn**
2 Tbsps. **mustard**

Instructions:
Boil the pasta in pure water with some salt and oil of choice, and strain it. Cut the veggies and the tuna. Mix all ingredients in a bowl and stir well.
Enjoy!

My notes:

Sweet Wholegrain Bread

Ingredients:
4 cups **water**
6-7 1/2 cups **buckwheat or millet flour**
1 1/2 cup **melted coconut butter**
1 1/2 cup **brown sugar or maple syrup**
2 cups **honey**
2 cups **molasses**
1/2 cup **soy milk powder**
1 tsp. **salt**
1 tsp. **cinnamon**
1 tsp. **nutmeg**
2 tsps. **baking powder**
Some **apricots, raisins, almonds, walnuts** (optional)

Instructions:
Mix all ingredients well. Knead the dough until everything is fully blended. Take a baking pan and cover it with vegetable oil and some flour (to avoid the bread from sticking to it). Spread the dough so that it is not thicker than half an inch. Bake the bread at 150 deg. C (300 F) for about an hour. Next, leave the bread in the oven and dry it at 50 deg. C (120 F) for 2 hours. Store the bread wrapped in a kitchen towel in a bread box.

Homemade Spinach Bread

Ingredients:
2 cups **wholegrain emmer or einkorn flour**
1-1 1/2 **cup water**
2 Tbsps. **dry yeast**
1 Tbsp. **maple syrup**
1 Tbsp. **salt**
2 fistfuls grated **hard cheese** (such as Gouda)
2 fistfuls **spinach**
Some **spices** according to your taste
Some **olive oil**

Instructions:
Use a sieve and sift the flour – do not leave any large particles in. Place the flour on the clean kitchen counter in a pile. Form a hole in the center and fill it with the yeast, the sugar, salt, and some water. Start mixing the ingredients forming the dough. Add more water to reach the consistency of soft dough. Knead the mixture until everything is fully homogenous. Place the dough in a bowl and cover it with a towel or wrapping foil. Let it sit for about 30 minutes.

In the meantime, boil the spinach with some salt for 3-5 minutes, strain it, and wash it gently with water. After the 30 minutes, the dough should have doubled its size. Now it is time to roll it out with the rolling pin. It should be about 0.2 inch (0.5 cm) thick. Take a baking pan, cover it with oiled paper and place half of the dough inside (we will cover the filling with the other half like a blanket).

Do not cut the dough. Grease it with some olive oil, put the cheese, the spinach and the spices in, and cover them with the other half of the dough. Tuck all ends of the bread so that the filling is fully covered. Grease the top of the bread with olive oil and sprinkle some spices. Leave the raw bread to rest a little bit while you start heating the oven. Place the bread on the heated oven at 180 deg. C (356 F) and bake for about 30 minutes.

Quick and Easy Fiber Beer Bread

Ingredients:
1 1/2 cup **wholegrain emmer or einkorn flour**
1/2 cup **ground flax seeds**
2 cups **"live" beer**
1 Tbsp. **baking powder**
1 tsp. **salt**
Several Tbsps. **olives** (without the kernels)
2 Tbsps. **herbs** according to your taste – rosemary, thyme, mint, etc.
2 Tbsps. **seeds** – pumpkin, sunflower, poppy, sesame seeds, etc.
Some **olive oil**

Instructions:

Note: the olives need to be as dry as possible – you can spread them on some kitchen paper to absorb the extra liquid.

Mix the flour, flax seeds, the baking powder, salt, the olives, and the herbs in a bowl. Stir well and slowly start pouring the beer in the mix. Use a fork to stir the mixture. The goal is to reach a semi-liquid consistency (like the one for cakes). Take a bread baking mold, cover it with the olive oil and pour the baking mixture in. Sprinkle the seeds on top. Bake the bread for 20 minutes in a preheated oven at 200 deg. C (390 F). Next, lower the temperature at 180 deg. C (356 F) and bake for 40-50 more minutes.

Corn & Pumpkin Bread

Ingredients:
2 cups **pumpkin**
1 cup **wholegrain emmer/einkorn flour**
1 1/2 cup **polenta** (cornmeal mush)
1 cup **green onion**
4 **eggs**
1 1/2 cup **milk**
2 Tbsps. maple **syrup/coconut sugar**
2 Tbsps. **baking powder**
8 Tbsps. **vegetable oil**
A pinch of **salt**

Instructions:

Peel the pumpkin, remove the seeds and grind it. Cut the onion in small pieces or mince it in a kitchen chopper. In a large bowl mix the polenta, the pumpkin, the onion, the flour, the sugar, salt, and the baking powder. Next, add the milk, the eggs, and the oil. Stir well to blend all ingredients. The result has to be a semi-liquid mixture.

Take a suitable baking mold and cover it with vegetable oil. Pour the mixture in and bake for 30 minutes at 200 deg. C (390 F). The oven has to be heated beforehand. Check if the bread is well baked – prick it with a toothpick and see if there is any dough stuck to it. If so, the bread needs more time to be fully cooked.

Aromatic Bread with Ginger and Molasses

Ingredients:
1 cup **wholegrain emmer/einkorn flour**
1/2 cup **ground flax seeds**
2 tsps. **baker's yeast**
1 1/2 tsp. **salt**
1/2 cup **water**
~1 cup cow/goat or vegetable **milk**
5 Tbsps. **molasses**
1 1/2 Tbsps. **olive or sunflower oil**
5 **clove buds**
1/2 tsp. grated **ginger root**
1 **cinnamon stick**

Instructions:

Place the water, the ginger, clove buds, and cinnamon in a pot and heat it. Let the infusion simmer for 3-5 minutes on low heat. Next, take it off the heat, cover it with a lid and let it cool off. Strain the mixture and add the milk to the decoction. Mix the flour, the flax seeds, and the yeast in a large bowl. Add all other ingredients stir slowly, cover the bowl with a lid or a kitchen foil, and leave the mixture for about 15 minutes for the yeast to start bulging. Next, start stirring the dough with a kitchen robot on medium for about 5-7 minutes. The goal is to reach a soft consistency, easy to knead and spread. Cover the dough and leave it to rest for 15 more minutes. Take a bread mold, grease it with some olive oil and place the dough inside. Leave the bread to rest one last time for 40 minutes. In the meantime, prepare the oven – heat it to 200 deg. C (390 F). Bake the bread for about 40-50 minutes until it is fully cooked.

My notes:

Sweet Bread with Dates

Ingredients:
1 1/2 cup **wholegrain emmer/einkorn flour**
1 1/2 tsp. **baker's yeast**
3 1/2 Tbsps. **butter**
1 cup **water**
1 tsp. **salt**
1/2 cup **dates**
Some **sesame seeds**

Instructions:
Warm the water and melt the butter to body temperature. Mix the yeast and the flour. Next, mix everything (except the dates and the sesame seeds) in a kitchen robot and stir on low for 2-3 minutes. Let the mixture rest for about 15 minutes. In the meantime remove the pits from the dates and cut the fruits in pieces. Add the dates to the mix and stir again for 5-7 minutes.

Take the dough and form it in a round ball. Cover it with oil and leave it in a warm room for an hour. Knead the dough every 15 minutes and cover it with a kitchen towel. Next, place the bread in a baking mold and cover it with the sesame seeds. Cover it again with the towel and leave it to rest for 30 more minutes.

Heat the oven at 220 deg. C (420 F) and bake the bread for about 20-25 minutes until it forms a nice golden crust.

Quick and Easy Oregano Wholegrain Bread Loaves

Ingredients:

1 kilo (4 cups) **wholegrain emmer/einkorn flour**

4 Tbsps. **Olive oil**

1/2 tsp. **baking soda**

2 Tbsps. **Fresh lemon juice or apple cider vinegar**

1/2 tsp. **ground sea or Himalayan salt**

2 Tbsps. **oregano**

Some **water**

Instructions:

In a large bowl mix the lemon juice and the baking soda. Next, add all other ingredients and mix. Add enough water to form a thick and sticky dough paste (like minced meat). Form small loaves with the desired shape and size. You can keep your hands moist for easier molding of the dough.

In the meantime prepare the oven – heat it to 220 deg. C (420 F).

Next, oil the baking pan and place the loaves in it. Make some cuts or pokes in them and place them in the oven. Bake for about 20 minutes until they form a nice brown crust. Take them out, sprinkle them with some pure water and cover them with a clean kitchen towel.

When they cool off completely, the loaves are ready for consumption!

Note: you can add whatever spices you like. You can even add some flax powder, or different seeds – sesame, sunflower, pumpkin, etc.

Easy Simple Wholegrain Bread

Ingredients:
1 kilo (4 cups) **wholegrain emmer/einkorn flour**
1 cup **water**
3 **eggs**
1 tsp. **baking soda**
Some **ground sea or Himalayan salt**
2-3 Tbsps. **Olive oil**

Instructions:
In a large bowl mix the flour, the baking soda, and the salt. In another container, mix the eggs, the water, and the olive oil. Whisk well until everything is fully homogenous. Next, add the egg mixture to the flour bowl and mix, you will reach nice and smooth kneadable dough. If it is too sticky, add more flour.

Next, take a baking pan and grease it with some olive oil. Place the dough inside and spread it thoroughly. Make some pokes with a fork all over the bread. Bake for about 35 minutes in a preheated oven at 200 deg. C (390 F).

Raw Mini Pizza

Ingredients:
1/2 cup **wholegrain emmer/einkorn flour**
1/2 cup **sprouted seeds** (sunflower, pumpkin, quinoa)
4 Tbsps. **Raw sesame seeds**
Some **Himalayan salt**
5 Tbsps. **Pure water**
4 Tbsps. **Raw cashews**
2 average **peppers**
2 pinches **turmeric powder**

Instructions:
Soak the cashews in some water for at least 2 hours. We will need them later.

Grind the sesame seeds and mix them with the sprouts, the wholegrain flour, the water and a little bit of salt. The goal is to reach dough that can be easily molded. Divide the mixture in several pieces and spread them to form the pizza crusts. Place them in a baking pan covered with oiled paper and bake them in the oven at 50 deg. C (120 F) for about 2 hours. If you have a dehydrator, you can use it as well. The crusts will become nicely crunchy.

Now it is time for the topping. Wash the soaked cashews thoroughly. Place them in a blender along with the peppers, turmeric powder, some salt and 5 Tbsps. water. Stir until you reach a nice homogenous consistency.

When the crusts are baked/dehydrated, simply cover them with the raw pesto. Voila!

5. Change the place you shop

Search for local producers. Their fruits and veggies are less likely to be treated with chemicals and artificial fertilizers. The same principle applies to meat – local farmers usually take better care of their animals – they are free range and usually not treated with hormones and antibiotics. It is easier to go to the place, get acquainted with the producers, and learn more about their methods of growing produce or animals. This is an excellent strategy to help your local community and to support eco and bio farmers.

6. Decrease your intake of addictive toxic substances

These substances include alcohol, recreational drugs, artificial food additives, etc. **Always consult with your doctor before making any changes with your prescription medications!** And search for a GP who supports natural healing practices. More and more physicians open to alternative and less harmful treatments. Here I am going to mention how grateful I am for finding my personal doctor! She is the perfect example of a medical professional who fully accepts and acknowledges the fact that we humans are creatures of Nature, and if we make healthy daily habits, artificial drugs won't be necessary, or they would be decreased drastically! Here I also must mention that I fully appreciate and respect the medical science and its huge progress serving mankind! But in many cases, if we change our lifestyle, our dietary habits, our physical activity, and manage stress levels, the need for strong and harsh drugs will be miniscule. And prevention is essential!

7. Quitting coffee and other caffeinated drinks

This may not seem very easy, but it is totally achievable. First of all, why cutting off coffee? There is a huge discussion on the pros and cons of drinking it. For me, there are a couple of things that tipped the scale towards the negative impact of this drink. Caffeine in very small quantities can stimulate the mind and give us a sense of energy rush. But becoming addicted to it, means that to sustain that energy level, we need more and more cups of coffee. Consequently, these high amounts of the stimulant dehydrate the body (we all know that nowadays most of us are chronically dehydrated), agitate the nervous system, overload the heart, increase the acidity in the cells, induce anxiety, raise the blood-pressure etc. So, if you have any type of condition connected to the above mentioned reasons, consider quitting coffee or decreasing its amounts as much as you can. If you are a heavy coffee addict, the "cold turkey" method can be extremely unpleasant experience. I used to drink just one espresso per day and it took me more than a month with severe headaches to withdraw from caffeine. So, it is best to try a more gentle incremental approach. For example, choose a healthy substitute (like ground coffee, chicory, tea, etc.) and start slowly decreasing the amount of coffee while increasing the natural substitute. If you drink 5 cups of coffee, try for a month to intake only 4 and the 5th should be the tea/ground coffee. Give your body enough time to get used to the change and adapt. When you feel ready, decrease the amount with one more cup of coffee, and substitute it with water, or other healthier option. Carbonated drinks are not advisable.

Another excellent substitute option for coffee is pure water mixed with freshly squeezed lemon juice. It instantly tones the body and helps with its morning cleansing processes. You can find more information about the numerous benefits of lemon water in the next chapters.

8. Quitting cigarettes

I am not sure if I can really help on this one, because I have never been a smoker myself. Nevertheless, the thing that comes to my mind is one book from which a lot of people gained great benefit. It's "Allen Carr's Easyway to Stop Smoking". The other thing about achieving anything in this life is to be committed, determined, and persistent. Sometimes there is a psychological barrier to quitting our bad habits, we need to identify and disempower. Maybe this is why this book is so helpful to many. Try different approaches, and don't give up, if you really want to quit this vice. If you do not wish to stop smoking, at least try to abstain from this habit for a period of time while you do a body detox. Many people report that after regular cleansing procedures and yoga, the body naturally starts to feel repulsed by cigarettes, alcohol, and other unhealthy substances. Keep the faith!

9. Natural cosmetics

Many of us know that most cosmetic products (even for babies) are packed with chemicals. Again, just like the food we eat, they contain preservatives, colorings, metals, parabens, petroleum derivatives, etc. It may seem like not a big deal, but it is. If we ingest a toxic substance, our bodies try their best to get rid of it ASAP. The hard-working liver and our kidneys will do most of the job. But what happens when the toxin goes through the skin? It enters directly into the blood stream! Given that the skin is our biggest organ, taking good care of it is essential. But fear not! Eco and bio industries are gathering speed and more and more toxin-free cosmetic treatments can be found on the market. There is also another option! Making your own SPA at home! Even if you are not very skillful and dexterous, you can find many ideas for your own custom easy to make cosmetics. Find some ideas in "Toxin-free Homemade Easy Beauty Recipes"

These were some of my suggestions on how to start making better, healthier, and toxin-free choices in everyday life. If you are hungry for more information about healthy holistic living, go to **http://mindbodyandspiritwellbeing.com**. All the information there is totally free! You will learn how to live a more healthy, energetic, conscious, and successful life.

Daily detoxing rituals

*D*etox doesn't have to be difficult or a tedious job. If you want to start cleansing your body slowly, there are many small habits that you can incorporate in your lifestyle. And they are fast and painless! Taking small, but consistent steps towards any goal is key for any success. So, daily habits, especially combined with slowly cutting down on the toxin intake, should not be underestimated. There is even a chance that you won't need anything else to purify your physique. These little techniques are very easy and doable and can make a huge difference in the long run.

1. Pranayama

The art of breathing – simply breathing can have an enormous impact on our health. Yogis know this fact and incorporated different breathing exercises in their daily practices. Of course, the quality of the air should not be overlooked. If you have access to purer air to breathe deeply, absolutely take advantage of it! If you live in a highly urbanized place, at least try to visit some sort of park where you can do Pranayama amongst the trees. Being closer to nature always has a beneficial impact on our bodies, minds and spirits. My grandparents come from a very small village in the beautiful mountains in Bulgaria. I can tell you, the place there is magical – the air is so fresh and energizing! No matter how tired I felt, one night of sound sleep in the village and I wake up full of vitality! Later on I realized it is the air that makes all the difference. And one more thing – most people living in these regions are centenarians!

Why breathing is so important? Because our lungs and heart are like communicating vessels – even a simple change in one of them will immediately reflect on the other, and vice versa. The heart pumps the blood, which carries the oxygen that we inhale through our lungs. So, if you have any type of condition related to the cardiovascular system - start doing Pranayama!

Here are some basic yoga breathing exercises that can help you detox your body on a daily basis. Remember that consistency is the key to success in every area of life! So, try to do them every day, or every other day.

    a. *Abdominal/diaphragm breathing* – I put this one first, because it is extremely powerful and beneficial. Start by focusing on the muscles of your abdomen and start breathing through the nose by expanding your belly. Your shoulders and chest should not be moving – you can even put one of your hands on the chest and the other – on your belly. Only the hand on the lower part of the body should be moving as you breathe. Repeat it as many times a day as you like, and as long as you feel comfortable. This exercise is excellent for relieving daily stress and soothing the nervous system.

    b. *High breathing* – this is the exact opposite of the previous one. This technique is very good for the lungs – it increases their capacity and has a cleansing effect. Lie down and again put one arm on the belly and the other one – on the chest. Inhale through the nose and feel how your lungs expand while the abdomen remains still. Exhale slowly, and consciously, and repeat as many times you feel you need to.

c. *Full/Complete breathing* – as the name suggests, here we are going to use the whole torso while breathing. So, as you slowly inhale, feel how fully you fill your body with air. Expand both the belly and the chest area. Again, breathe deeply and slowly, and focus your attention on the movement of the air through your body. This exercise alone can give you a huge energetic boost as well as a deep cellular cleanse! Most of the time our breathing is pretty shallow, which limits the supply of oxygen, vital for the cells and our overall wellbeing.

As you master these techniques you can start measuring your breath. For example, inhale as you count to 3, hold your breath for 3 seconds, and exhale slowly for 3 seconds. As you progress, you can stretch the numbers and keep exercising the lungs, and expanding their capacity. Daily breath exercises are fast and free, but priceless!

2. Visualization

You can even make a step further and include the enormous power of our imagination. As you do your daily breathing exercises, start visualizing! As you inhale, imagine pure light and divine energy filling every cell of your being, imagine yourself shining and radiating like a star. As you exhale, visualize all negativity and toxicity leaving your physical temple and dissolving into space. The power of such mental exercises should not be underestimated. Our imagination is linked to our sub-consciousness, which is responsible for all our autopilot functions – breathing, coordination, heartbeat, hormone secretion, and cleansing. We do not consciously do all these things, our mind would become overwhelmed. So, all these vital actions are being taken care of by the sub-consciousness. This part of our mind does not understand words, but visual and emotional stimuli. This is why imagining how with each breath the body is purified, gives clear instructions to the sub-conscious mind to boost and activate this process. In other words, visualizing how your body is detoxed will multiply the effect of Pranayama and all other cleansing techniques you apply!

3. Sweat these toxins off!

This technique is fairly easy and you most probably already used it many times. It's plain sweating. As I said previously, our skin is a very important organ and has many vital functions. One of them is taking out as much harmful substances as possible. This is why when we go through some detox programs (even fasting), we get rashes, pimples, even itchy spots – this is our skin flushing out what's not good for the body. We can use this important auto cleansing function in daily life (or as often as we wish) to our advantage. There is nothing special about it – every time sweat come out of the glands, it carries out toxins with itself. What we can do is to help the process. One way to do this is to exercise – cardio trainings usually result in heavy sweating. If you can put on some extra clothing without feeling uncomfortable, the effect will be even greater. Another more pleasant option is to go to a sauna. The high temperature induces the natural body reflex to protect itself from overheating by perspiration.

A word of caution: intense cardio exercises as well as high-temperature saunas increase the heart rate and blood pressure. If you have any cardio vascular issues (especially hypertension), these techniques might not be suitable for you. Always consult with your physician before making such changes in your lifestyle.

4. Oil pulling

This is a very interesting daily cleansing technique. Actually it is dedicated to improving one's oral health, but it turns out that it has a detoxing effect on the whole body as well. First, I am going to describe it – it is very simple and easy. This procedure is executed first thing in the morning, before you wash your teeth, drink or eat anything. You are going to need some sort of cold pressed oil – sesame, coconut, virgin olive oil, sunflower seed, pumpkin seed, etc. You can enhance this procedure by adding a few drops of essential oils. For example, Tea tree oil - a natural antibiotic, which kills the bacteria accumulated in the mouth, and fights gum diseases. Another excellent option is Cinnamon – it also has strong antiseptic and antiviral properties, plus it tastes much better than Tea tree. Clove essential oil is perfect for the oral hygiene – it not only fights the bacteria, but also works as a local anesthetic (if you have any toothaches or wounds in the mouth, choose this essential oil until you visit the dentist/doctor).

Peppermint and Lemon essential oils are great for achieving fresh breath.

So, take a tablespoonful of the cold pressed oil, add a few drops of the desired essential oil, and start swishing it in your mouth – just like you do with a regular mouthwash. Do not even think about swallowing it! Keep "pulling" the oil as much as you can. The goal is to reach 20 min, but it may be difficult to be done right away. Start with whatever period of time feels appropriate and doable for you. As you build this habit and get used to the procedure, you can expand this time period. At first you may even feel nausea, but it will pass as you continue to apply this technique day in day out. Next, spit the oil into the trash – you may notice the substance had become whiter and thicker – this is good, this is what we aim for! After that, rinse your mouth thoroughly with water. You can rinse it with salty water afterwards if you wish to achieve even better disinfection (especially if you have sensitive teeth). That's it!

Notice how your teeth become much whiter in just a couple of days! This is a clear sign the oil had pulled out a lot of plaque. But it does much more than that. Our bodies try to take all unnecessary and harmful agents out through all possible outlets – urine, feces, sweat, pus, and mucus. They produce mucus, which had accumulated lots of bacteria, viruses, toxins, and so on, all the time in order to self-clean – through the nose, the lungs, the vulva, etc. The oil that we swish pulls this phlegm full of toxins out and thus, helping our bodies detox much easier and faster. Even though it seems a bit eccentric, this technique comes from ancient

Ayurveda and had been proven effective through the ages.

5. Pure water

Body detox does not have to be rocket science. Actually, all we do here is finding and implementing ways to help our corpus clean and heal itself. The main mechanism that it uses to flush out all unnecessary compounds is very simple – water. The liquid we intake nurtures the cells and takes out the wastes through the excretory system. Unfortunately, we tend to forget that. One side of the problem is that drinking water hasn't been formed as a habit. The other side is that most foods and drinks we intake make us even more dehydrated. They are dry, salty, sugary, with a lot of artificial preservatives, colorings, etc. Healthy pieces of advice are blasting from everywhere: *"Drink more water!"*, *"Drink more water!"*, *"Drink more water!"*. And usually the result is not very significant. Why? Because of the two main reasons I mentioned – we haven't established it as a habit, and we keep dehydrating ourselves. Have you even made a commitment such as *"From tomorrow I am going to drink the optimum daily amount of water!"* What happens next? What happened to me when I tried to achieve this goal is going to the bathroom every 5 min. It's certainly not very pleasant and convenient! I kept repeating this with little success throughout the years. Then it dawned on me – the body is not used to so much liquid, it does not know what to do with it! So, it either flushes it out immediately, or stores it making you look puffy. In other words, learning to drink more water comes hand in hand with eliminating dehydrating foods and liquids, and incrementally including more auqa in our diet. Another good option for us to consider is to make the water taste better. We have grown used to drinking all kinds of juices and beverages, that we have forgotten the pure taste of water. So, here are some examples:

a. **Water with lemon** – we will discuss this in detail later;

b. **Water with wheat grass powder** – it has extremely beneficial healing, and cleansing nutrients;

c. **Tea** – natural herbal water infusions are a great way to start drinking more water. Plus, they have many healing properties. Later, we will pay more attention to herbal teas.

Drinking water first thing in the morning has more benefits than you expect. It not only creates a feeling of fullness of the stomach, but it improves the whole organism. The same rule applies for bedtime when our bodies prepare for a good night rest. But why is it so important to start the day with a refreshing cup of pure water? It's simple – these are the hours in which the excretory organs (kidneys and intestines) work extra hard to cleanse the body. If we do not supply the necessary fluid, they cannot do their job properly. All the water that we intake in the morning is used to cleanse our organism and it is taken out immediately. It is best to use fresh pure clean water. In the next section, I will point out numerous ways on how to make this precious fluid healthier and cleaner. Use tap water as a last resort and add some lemon juice, honey or apple cider vinegar to neutralize the unwanted compounds in it. This may be the easiest and simplest detox method everyone can apply immediately, even the busiest person! It also accelerates our metabolic processes, delivering oxygen and nutrients to the cells of the body. If you are chronically dehydrated, start small. Your body will quickly get used to this new procedure. The optimum quantities are at least 2 cups of warm or lukewarm water right after getting out of bed and 2-3 more cups two hours later. But always listen to your body and adjust the amounts according to your needs and your daily schedule. Increase your daily water consumption slowly until you feel comfortable to the new amounts.

Why should we drink water (especially hot water or tea) in the morning on an empty stomach? Even gastroenterologists acknowledge the benefits of starting the day with a cup of hot water. As I already mentioned, during the night as we sleep, our bodies can finally have some quality time cleansing themselves. Mucus, food debris, and gastric juice start to accumulate on the walls of the gastrointestinal tract. When we take a cup of hot water in the morning, we help our bodies flush out all these toxic agents. This is why this hot liquid causes a gentle laxative effect – it's an automatic cleansing reaction. But that's not all! This warm beverage softens and loosens the gallbladder and excess bile leaves our bodies preventing us from gallstones formation.

How warm or hot should the morning water be? The best temperature for this cleansing procedure is between 30 and 40 degrees Celsius (86-104 degrees Fahrenheit). You don't want your beverage to be cool, nor too hot. Cold water is definitely not suitable for this morning ritual – it will only shock the body and irritate the gastrointestinal tract.

For people with more sensitive stomachs cold water may even cause severe diarrhea.

These beneficial effects can only be achieved on an empty stomach. Drinking water after a meal not only does not have any healthy consequences, but it could even do us harm. When we drink liquids during or after we intake food, we dilute the gastric juices and hinder digestion itself. On the contrary, water taken about half an hour before a meal, hydrates the stomach and prepares it for the proper break down of food.

If it's difficult for you to drink large quantities of water, do not despair! One cup warm water taken regularly in small sips is quiet enough to obtain its therapeutic effects. Remember to use only pure water (or suitable herbal tea) for this purpose. Other liquids like coffee, carbonated drinks, or artificial juices will not cause this healthy cleansing effect.

Healthy types of pure water

Water intake plays an essential part in detoxing our bodies. It hydrates our cells, enabling them to work properly and effectively, and taking all unnecessary compounds out through the urine and sweat. Most people pay attention to the quantities they drink every day, but there is one more thing we need to consider – the quality of the fluid. It is a well-known fact that in most parts of the world tap water is polluted. It may contain traces of the toxic chemicals, chlorine, scale, debris from old pipes, fluoride, etc. Consider yourself very lucky if your tap water is clean and safe to drink. But if you have any suspicions, take a moment to think about filtering and cleansing the most important fluid in our lives. There are many options available for you to try and decide which one works best for you. Or you can combine several options. I will list a few ideas right here:

a. *Pitcher (or other similar device) with replaceable filters* – inexpensive and effective way to purify your water. The active charcoal filters remove most of the Chlorine, pesticides, volatile organic substances, and improves the taste and quality of the liquid;

b. *Reverse osmosis home purifying systems* – it is much more expensive, but its effectiveness is greater – it removes about 99% of the Chlorine, bacteria, viruses, heavy metals, Fluoride, pesticides, radioactive substances, etc.

c. *Water distiller* – distilled water is widely discussed whether it is healthy or not. But for short periods of time annually it can gently cleanse the body, especially for people with a predisposition to kidney stones;

d. *Ice water* – it is fairly easy to prepare ice water at home. Fill a container about 2/3 of its capacity with water and put it in the freezer. When the water starts to freeze, remove the ice crust at the top (it contains deuterium), and put the container back in the freezer. When about 2/3 of the liquid is frozen, take it out and remove the remaining water. The remaining ice is your ice water. Drink the melted water in the next 5 hours. This procedure takes some time, but it is worth it – ice water stimulates the metabolism, and helps our bodies recover much easily. This water is not suitable for cooking;

e. ***Boiled water*** – a cup of boiled water on an empty stomach can make a huge difference in your health. It gently cleanses the body, soothes the nervous system, lowers the cholesterol levels, heals chronic constipation, prevents from all kinds of cardiovascular diseases, and many more;

f. ***Magnetized water*** – magnet therapy is very popular with its healing effects on our bodies. We can use the same principles for the water we drink. Just take a magnetic therapy bracelet and put it around a bottle of water for about an hour, and the magnetic water is ready. This liquid can benefit your liver and kidneys – dissolves kidney stones and gallstones. It can also remove cholesterol plaques, and can lower the blood sugar level. Soothes the digestive tract, various skin issues, and it can even decrease the hair loss.

g. ***Zeolite (Clinoptilolite)*** – this is a magical mineral – one of the few, which are negatively charged (this means it connects to heavy metals, toxins, radioactive particles, phosphates, ammonia etc. and neutralizes them). It contains lots of important elements for our health – Calcium, Potassium, Sodium, and more. The benefits of using Zeolite as a water filter are numerous – it cleanses the body and promotes weight loss, improves digestion, soothes the high blood pressure, insomnia, heavy perspiration, stress, it's a strong anti-oxidant, cleanses the kidneys and prevents from kidney stones formation, lowers the chances of developing cancer, stimulates the immune system, and many more. **Use only pure high quality Zeolite, which had been refined, and all impurities had been removed!**

So, how to prepare your clean healthy Zeolite water? Put about 100 gr pure Clinoptilolite lumps in a large container with 5 liters mineral water. Let them sit for at least 8 hours, and your Zeolite water is ready. It is advisable to drink more water daily because this mineral has distinct cleansing effects. You can drink only Zeolite water or combine it with the one you usually consume. When you finish the 5 liters, just refill the container and wait 8 more hours. The Clinoptilolite will hold its healing properties for about 3 months, after that you will need to change it.

h. *Ionized and alkalized water* – this type of water is often called "live", because it is energetically charged, and for its numerous healing powers. Regular consumption of ionized water can significantly improve your health – it alkalizes the body (you know cancer cells develop only in acid environment), detoxifies, energizes, boosts the metabolism, improves digestion, strengthens the immune system, promotes weight loss, and much more. Most brands enhance this liquid with Magnesium, which makes it even healthier.

6. Morning lemon water purifier

Now that we know how to clean the water we drink, we can use it with other natural detoxing agents for optimum results. Lemon is the perfect example! First thing in the morning (when our bodies cleanse themselves) drink a glass of this magical potion. It is very easy to prepare – just mix a glass of lukewarm pure water with freshly squeezed lemon juice. Keep in mind that if the water is too warm, it may destroy most of the citrus' vitamins. If you feel inspired to boost this detox drink even more, include some fresh grated ginger. Excess fat cells will have no other option, but to leave the body! And you will have stronger immune system, fewer inflammations, better digestion, more energy, and so on.

There are a lot of reasons to include lemon water in our diets. Although it looks like a fairly simple technique, it should not be underestimated. Here are some the benefits of this detoxifying liquid:

a. ***Warm water with lemon helps the digestion.*** Its chemical compositions are very similar to our saliva and stomach juices. The citric acid in lemons interacts with the enzymes and other acids in the digestive system, which stimulates the secretion of gastric fluids. This makes the breakdown of the food much easier.

b. ***Helps the work of the liver.*** Lemon juice is extremely valuable for liver cleansing. It is no coincidence that most liver detox programs include freshly squeezed lemon juice diluted in water. The sour beverage stimulates the enzyme secretion of our biggest internal organ, helps it take out the toxins and flushes them out of the body through the excretory system.

c. ***Fights constipation.*** If you use warm water with lemon, you can help one of most important organs regarding body cleansing and our overall health – the intestines and the colon. If you have irregular bowels, consider including warm lemon water in your diet immediately. After all, what is the point of trying to cleanse our organism, if we cannot take out the trash properly?

d. ***Lemons are powerful antioxidants.*** Regular consumption of this citrus water has a greater beneficial effect than we suspect – it regulates our metabolism (who wants a slender body?), flushes out cholesterol plaques from the blood vessels, protects us from free radicals and slows down the aging process. This citrus fruit is the living proof that health and beauty go hand in hand!

e. ***Lemons contain high quantities of Potassium.*** But why do we need this mineral? Potassium is an extremely important compound for our bodies – together with Sodium, they work as powerful neurotransmitters. In other words, we need these essential chemicals for a healthy and strong nervous system. The neurons in our bodies need sufficient amount of Potassium in order to sustain the proper communication between the brain and the heart (and the overall cardiovascular system). If you want to maintain perfect heart health, regular intake of this mineral is a must. Low Potassium levels may cause depression, anxiety, brain fog, and even fear.

f. Moreover, with a single glass of water mixed *with fresh lemon juice, you supply your cells with Calcium and Magnesium.* We all know how important Calcium is for the proper care for our bones, preventing from rickets and osteoporosis. Magnesium is another underestimated, but essential mineral for our health. It is indispensable for the heart and the nervous system.

g. We are not done with this precious yellow fruit, yet! Lemons also contain various vitamins such as Carotene (~0.01 mg), Vitamin B1 (~0.04 mg), Vitamin B2 (~0.02 mg), Vitamin B5 (~0,2 mg), Vitamin B6 (~0.06 mg), Vitamin C (~40-70 0 mg), Vitamin PP (~0.1 mg). As I already mentioned this citrus fruit can offer important minerals like Calcium, Potassium, Magnesium, Phosphorus, Sodium, and Iron.

h. Taken daily, the water-lemon mixture can help lower the blood pressure. The early stages of hypertension (if the blood pressure does not rise above 160/90) can be treated with fresh lemon juice. For the first 2-3 weeks, squeeze 2 lemons a day. When the tension starts to drop, reduce the dosage to 1 lemon daily. *Always consult with your physician before making any changes in your medications!*

i. Reduces the acidity of the body. Nowadays it is a well-known fact that high acidity in our cells creates an excellent environment for the development of various diseases, viruses, and bacteria. Drinking lemon water before each meal (especially if the meal will cause a drop in our pH levels), can restore the alkalinity in our bodies. Most people are confused by the sour taste of lemons and consider them as acidic, but this is not true. When digested in our stomachs, citrus fruits have an alkaline reaction.

j. **Indispensable for people with gout and various joint issues.** Lemon water has an extremely favorable effect on our joints, because it dilutes the uric acid in the organism. As we know, when there are excess amount of this acid, and the body cannot take it all out, it stores it mainly in the joints and muscles, causing serious problems. Taking lemon water and combining it with a proper diet plan can make a tremendous difference in those people's health!

k. **Reduces mucus secretion.** The huge amount of Vitamin C in this precious fruit can improve our digestion, boost our immunity, and cleanse our body from excess mucus. This is extremely valuable for people experiencing problems with their lungs (asthma, bronchitis and so on). During the night as we are sleeping, our bodies do not stop working. On the contrary, there are a lot of intense processes happening during our rest time. One of these major operations is cleansing. The stomach accumulates as much toxins and mucus as it can and prepares them to be flushed out first thing in the morning. This is why we may have unpleasant morning breath, sputa coming from the lungs (especially for smokers), excess mucus from the eyes and nose, etc. In other words, during the first hours of the day our bodies try to dispose of all unnecessary substances accumulated all night. When we drink lemon water before breakfast on an empty stomach, we accelerate and assist this important cleansing process. If we wish to boost this detox, we can add one more cup of this citrus beverage with one tablespoon of raw honey half an hour before bedtime. With these two simple steps we have accomplished more than we could imagine!

l. *Excellent coffee substitute.* Previously I have already mentioned that lemon water can be used in the morning instead of the black refreshing beverage. If you are determined to break from your caffeine dependency, this healthier alternative is an excellent choice! It will tone your body, but unlike coffee, it won't deprive you of essential nutrients and it won't dehydrate you!

m. *Assists the weight loss.* I am completely aware that most people start detoxing for the main purpose of achieving slimmer body. And that's perfectly fine. Many weight loss plans start with lemon water on an empty stomach. But why is that? Citric acid speeds our metabolism and helps us break down fat tissues more easily. Lemons also contain some amounts of pectin, which normalizes the blood sugar levels, and last but not least – cleanses the lymph and helps its proper flow. One more important fact, the sour juice from the lemon stimulates the work of the liver – it starts to increase the bile secretion along with toxins and mucus it had accumulated, and the water flushes these harmful agents out through the excretory organs. So, start your day with a cup of warm water mixed with lemon juice, but wait for at least half an hour before having breakfast for the beverage to do its magic! To maximize your weight loss results, take a cup of this healthy mixture half an hour before each meal – it will speed the metabolism, start melting the extra fat, and the containing pectin will reduce your appetite. If you are counting your calories intake, consider that lemons have as low as 31 kcal per 100 grams.

Here is another great *recipe for body cleansing and weight loss*. Make a simple green tea water infusion (pour hot water onto some green tea leaves and let it sit for a few minutes), then add some Apple Cider Vinegar and a slice of lemon. Increase the consumption of fresh fruits and vegetables, have more salads dressed with virgin olive oil and lemon juice and choose your preferred type of regular exercise. And that's it!

Do you want a gentler version? Simply add some raw honey in your lemon water. *Make sure the liquid is not hotter than your body temperature (to keep all the good stuff in the honey).*

Whew! So many benefits in such a small fruit! But let me add a few words on how to prepare this cleansing fluid. First of all, try to use as pure water as possible. I have already mentioned some techniques on how to purify your water. But if you are short on time, store bought mineral water will do. Warm the water and add freshly squeezed lemon juice. If you wish to add some raw honey, make sure the temperature of the liquid is not higher than the body temperature (to protect all nutrients, vitamins, and minerals in it).

Important note! Every time you eat citrus fruits (in this case lemons) or drink citrus juice, rinse your mouth afterwards. You can rinse it with plain water or you can add some salt. Do not brush the teeth, just rinse them! The acid in these fruits can damage the enamel and can cause tooth decay or sensitivity. The same rule applies also to all kinds of vinegar! If you wish to brush the teeth, wait at least half an hour before doing so.

Another important thing to consider regarding regular lemon consumption! If you eat lemons or drink their juice on an empty stomach, your stomach may have a unpleasant reaction. The citric acid stimulates the secretion of gastric fluids and people with sensitive stomachs, gastritis, pancreatitis, cholecystitis, hepatitis, enterocolitis, heartburn, ulcers or any kind of diseases of the bile ducts will have to avoid consuming lemons before meals. If you are one of those people, it is advisable for you to try other gentler types of detoxification!

Also, if you decide to end your day with a nice cup of warm water/tea with lemon juice, make sure you do it at least an hour before you go to sleep. Lemons are packed with nutrients, vitamins, and minerals that can stimulate the nervous system, which can prevent you from falling asleep easily.

Should you have any kinds of chronic illnesses or any concerns about your personal detox program, do not hesitate to consult with your physician!

7. Detox tea/drinks

It is hard for some people to increase the amount of water they drink. I believe most of us feel that way – we are so used to drinking something that has a particular taste. If you are one of those people, do not worry! As the saying goes: *Every problem can become an opportunity!* That's what we are going to do here! We can combine the natural detox effect of water and amplify it with the irreplaceable assistance of herbs. Some plants have the ability to purify our cells, help them flush out the toxins, and fight against free radicals. Plus, they tend to slow down aging! Here are some herbs known to have those beneficial effects – Green tea, Licorice, Neem, Dandelion, Milk Thistle, Turmeric, Wormwood, Manjistha, Cilantro, Peppermint/Spearmint, Eucalyptus, Stinging nettle, and many more. Find the ones that taste good to you and are available in your area. You may find pre-made detox herbal teas on the market – they are so many choices available right now. Don't forget the fact that herbs are natural detox sources, but that does not mean they should be underestimated. Consult with your physician before taking any herbal remedies or supplements.

Here are some nice refreshing, detoxing, strengthening and healing herbal infusions you can prepare at home instead of the usual coffee:

Aromatic Tea with Milk and Spices

Ingredients:
2 cups **pure water**

1 Tbsp. **tea** or **herb** of choice

1 Tbsp. **coconut sugar** or Grade B maple syrup

4-5 grains **cardamom**

4-5 **clove buds**

1 **cinnamon stick**

2 **stars anise**

1 cup **vegetable milk** (almond, soy, oat, etc.)

Instructions:
Bring the water to boil and take it off the heat. Add the herbs, sugar, spices, and the milk. Cover the pot with a lid and let the ingredients steep for some time. Strain the infusion and enjoy!

My notes:

Sea Buckthorn Tea Blend

Ingredients:
2-3 cm (~ 1 inch) **ginger root**
100 grams (~ 7 Tbsps.) **Sea Buckthorn fruits** (Hippophae)
2 **cinnamon sticks**
2 **orange segments**
Several **fresh Mint leaves**
500 ml (2 cups) **boiling water**
Some **honey**

Instructions:
Peel and grate the ginger root. Mash the Sea Buckthorn fruits and the orange. Mix the puree with the ginger. Divide the mixture in 2 parts and place them in appropriate tea cups. Put a cinnamon stick and a couple of Mint leaves in each cup as well. Pour the hot water in the cups and let the infusion steep for several minutes. Strain the mixture and when the tea reaches body temperature, add the honey. Enjoy!

My notes:

Black Tea with Cranberries

Ingredients:
3 1/2 cups **water**

1/4 cup **brown/coconut sugar or maple syrup**

1 cm (1/2 inch) **ginger root**

2 **clove buds**

2 tea bags **Black tea**

1/2 cup **cranberry juice**

2 Tbsps. **lemon juice**

1 **cinnamon stick**

1 **anise star**

Instructions:
Put the water, sugar, anise, ginger, cinnamon, and clove in a metal pot. Heat the mixture until it starts to boil. Remember to stir. Let the infusion simmer for 2 minutes and take it off the heat. Put the tea bags in the liquid and let them steep for 10 minutes. Next, take them out, strain the infusion, and add the lemon and cranberry juices. Stir well and serve!

My notes:

Black Tea with Citruses

Ingredients:
2 cups **freshly brewed black tea**
1 **lime**
1 **orange**
2 Tbsps. **honey**
1/2 tsp. **cinnamon**

Instructions:
Wash the citruses thoroughly and cut them in pieces (with the zest). Cover them with the cinnamon and pour the tea on top. Let the mixture steep for about 5 minutes. When the infusion cools to body temperature, add the honey and stir.

Moroccan Tea

Ingredients:
1-2 **cinnamon sticks**
4 **clove buds**
Orange or lemon zest
Some **ginger powder**
1 **lime**
A bunch of **Spearmint**
3 tsps. **black tea**
2 cups **water**
Some **coconut sugar, maple syrup or honey**

Instructions:

Cut the citrus zests in thin strips. Grind or mince the Mint leaves and cut the lime in pieces. Mix all ingredients in a large pot. Bring the water to boil and pour it onto the herbs and spices. Let them steep for 5-7 minutes. Strain the infusion and sweeten it with the desired sugary product.

Immune Boosting Tea Blend

Ingredients:
1 tea bag **Peppermint**
1 cup **hot water**
1 1/2 tsp. **grated ginger root**
1/8 tsp. **turmeric**
1/8 tsp. **cinnamon**
1 Tbsp. **honey**
A pinch of **black pepper**

Instructions:

Soak the tea bag in the hot water. Cover the cup with a lid and let the herb steep for 2-3 minutes. Add all spices (ginger, turmeric, cinnamon, and pepper) to the infusion and stir. Let the mixture cool off to body temperature and strain it. Add the honey and the tea is ready!

Healing Anti-Cough Tea

Ingredients:
1 tea bag **green tea**
1 cup **hot water**
1/2 tsp. **ground clove buds**
1/2 tsp. **turmeric**
1/2 tsp. **dry Thyme**
2 tsps. **honey**
1 **lemon**

Instructions:
Place the green tea, the clove powder, the turmeric, and the thyme in a bowl or a cup. Pour the hot water in and place the lid on. Let the herbs soak nicely.

In the meantime, squeeze the juice from the lemon.

When the infusion cools off, strain it and add the honey and the lemon juice.

Hot Winter Tea for Colds and the Flu

Ingredients:
2 cups **hot water**
1/2 tsp. **chili pepper powder**
1 Tbsp. **black tea**
2-3 Tbsps. **Fruit juice** of choice

Instructions:

Put the tea in a large cup or a pot and pour the hot water in. Cover it with a lid and let it steep for a couple of minutes. Strain the tea and, add the chili powder and the fruit juice. Stir and drink!

Note: if you have a sensitive stomach, or any other type of illness in the gastrointestinal tract (gastritis, ulcers, colitis, hemorrhoids, etc.), this tea might not be suitable for you. Consult with a doctor beforehand!

Detoxing Ayurvedic Tea

Ingredients:
1/4 tsp. **cumin seeds**
1/4 tsp. **coriander seeds**
1/4 tsp. **dry fennel**
2 cups **water**
A slice of **lemon** (optional)
Some **honey** (optional)

Instructions:

Heat the water to the boiling point. Add the spices, cover the pot with the lid and let the herbs steep. When the infusion cools off to body temperature, strain it. Add the lemon and the honey, if you desire.

Dairy Tea with Spices

Ingredients:
2 Tbsps. **grated ginger root**
1 1/2 cup bio goat/cow milk or vegetable **milk**
1/2 cup **water**
1/3 tsp. **cinnamon**
A few **green cardamom grains**
A pinch of **grated nutmeg**
1 Tbsp. **honey or maple syrup**
1/3 tsp. **black tea**

Instructions:
Bring the water to boil and add the ginger. In about a minute, add the milk, the spices, and the tea. Let the decoction simmer for 5-7 minutes on very low heat. Next, take the tea off the heat and let it cool off. Strain the infusion and when the tea reaches body temperature, add the honey.

Healthy Pine Tips Tea

Ingredients:
2 liters (8 cups) **pure water**
1 cup **pine tips**
Some **honey**
Some **lemon juice**

Instructions:

Wash the needles and place them in metal pot with the water. Heat the water and let the ingredients simmer for 7-8 minutes. Take the pot off the heat, cover it with the lid and let it cool off to body temperature. Strain the infusion, add the honey, the lemon juice, and enjoy!

Healthy Calendula Tea

Ingredients:
1 1/2 cup **pure water**
10 fresh **Calendula blossoms**
1 tsp. **green tea**
2 tsps. **Ginger root**
1 **cinnamon stick**

Instructions:

Wash and wipe dry the blossoms carefully. Next, pluck off the petals. Next, peel and grind the ginger root. Place it in a metal pot, pour the water in, and heat it on the stove. Let the ginger simmer for 5 minutes. Next, put the Calendula petals, the green tea, and the cinnamon stick in a pot and cover them with the ginger infusion. Let the herbs steep for at least 15 minutes, and strain the tea.

If you wish to sweeten the beverage, wait until it reaches body temperature and add some honey.

Rosehips & Apple Tea

Ingredients:
2 cups **green apples**
5 Tbsps. **dry rosehips**
4 cups **water**
1 **bio orange/lemon**
Some **honey**

Instructions:
Peel the apples, remove the seeds and cut them in pieces. Crush or mince the rosehips. Place the fruits in a metal pot and pour the water in. Heat the mixture and bring it to boil. Next, take the pot off the heat and let it cool off a little bit. Then, strain the infusion. Peel the orange or lemon and grate the zest. Add the grated skin to the tea and stir. When the liquid cools to body temperature, add the honey and stir again to melt it completely.

Rosehips Tea for Any Thyme (pun intended!)

Ingredients:
10 **rosehips**
5 **Thyme leaves**
1 Tbsp. **honey**
1 cup **water**

Instructions:

Put the water in a metal pot and heat it until it starts to boil. In the meantime grind or crush the rosehips. When the water is boiling put the rosehips in and let them simmer for 5 minutes. Next, add the Thyme and take the pot off the heat. Cover it with the lid and let the herbs steep for 10 more minutes. Strain the infusion and leave it to cool off to body temperature. Add the honey and stir.

Ginger and Anise Tea

Ingredients:
1 slice **lemon**
10 slices **fresh ginger root**
1 Tbsp. **honey**
Some **anise stars**
1 cup **water**

Instructions:

Place the ginger, the lemon and the anise in a cup and pour the hot water. If you do not like anise, you can substitute it with cinnamon. Cover the cup and let it steep for 10-15 minutes. Strain the mixture, and when the tea reaches body temperature, add the honey.

Refreshing Hibiscus Tea

Ingredients:
4 cups **water**
3 Tbsps. **Hibiscus**
10 dry **rosehip fruits**
1/2 **orange**
Some **honey**

Instructions:
Place the water and the plants in a metal pot and heat it. Let them simmer for about 3 minutes. Let the infusion cool off and strain it. Add the honey and some freshly squeezed orange juice.

Here are some more easy example recipes with herbs, plants, fruits, and veggies for detox, anti-aging, stronger immune system, and faster metabolism:

> a. *Anti-aging and cancer prevention detox potion:*
>
> You will need some grated ginger, 1 tsp. turmeric, some fresh mint leaves, and 500 ml (~17 o.z.) pure water. Bring the water to boil and add all ingredients. Stir for about 5 min, take the mixture off the heat, and strain. You can put some honey for sweetness, but you will have to wait until the liquid cools down to body temperature.

b. *Metabolism activation purifier:*

Bring 1 cup of clean filtered or mineral water to boil. Pour the hot liquid on 2 cloves of garlic (minced) and 1 tsp. cayenne pepper powder. Let it sit until the infusion is drinkable. This recipe is not suitable for people suffering from gastritis, stomach ulcers, and other gastric issues. Consult with your doctor first.

c. *Antioxidant detox teas:*

Pour 200 ml (~7 o.z.) hot pure water onto some dry Green tea herbs. Let it sit for about 10 min and strain. When the infusion cools to room temperature, add some freshly quizzed lemon juice and some raw honey.

d. *Fat burning cleansing potion:*

As I already mentioned, body toxicity is tightly related to fat storage. If our corpus could not manage to flush out all harmful compounds, it disarms them by embracing them with fat tissue. This recipe aims to help the body detoxify and naturally get rid of the extra weight. Take 200 ml (~7 o.z.) water and heat it. Next, add 1 tsp. cinnamon powder and let the mixture sit until it becomes lukewarm. Add some lemon juice and enjoy!

e. *Liver detox juice:*

The liver is one of the most important organs when it comes to detoxification. In the next book I will concentrate in many liver cleansing techniques. But here I am just going to mention one quick and easy recipe, suitable for daily use. You can take this tea for about a month's period. Boil a pinch of Milk Thistle in 200 ml water for a couple of minutes. Let it cool to room temperature and strain the infusion. You can add some coconut milk and honey according to your taste.

8. Yoga

Yoga is not just stretching the body and muscles or chanting mantras. Yoga is a holistic practice, which encompasses many different activities. Its benefits are more than you expect. Most people think that yoga is meant only to increase your flexibility. But this is just a drop in the ocean of health benefits of this ancient practice. Yes, if you regularly exercise yoga poses you will strengthen your muscles, ligaments and bones. But these visible effects are merely on the surface. You will be surprised how much yoga can do for you – physically, mentally, emotionally, and even spiritually. Take a look!

a. Improves digestion

A proper healthy diet with lots of fresh fruits and vegetables (with a lot of fiber) is crucial for our health and especially for our digestive system. But regular yoga practices can give us tremendous improvements in this area, too. There are many asanas (including the special internal organ massages), which target these important body systems. These poses help us improve the blood flow through these tissues and thus helping with our healthy digestion. And as we know, the easier and more effortlessly the digestion works, the more energy we have. And the more the body will be able to dedicate time and energy for its natural cleansing processes.

b. Fights the feeling of hunger

Most body cleansing procedures involve abstaining from food for a period of time. The feeling of hunger inevitably emerges and gives us discomfort. Fortunately, regular yoga practices can gradually build our physical and mental resistance against temptation. A study by the American Dietetic Association found that yoga is directly related to conscious eating. This positive effect comes from the full awareness when executing the asanas – it creates a strong connection between the body and the soul. We begin to recognize which foods are good for our bodies at the moment and when is the right time to eat. I see evidence of this study all around me. More and more people acknowledge that after a long period of regularly doing yoga, they naturally and gradually change their attitude towards the food they intake. Some start to feel even repelled from junk food and meat products.

c. Improves the brain function

You may already know that the most types of sports and exercises improve brain function through improving the blood flow to our heads. But yoga is special – it gives us real psychological benefits, too. The perfect combination of movement (mostly isometric) and conscious breathing can tremendously improve our ability to concentrate and relax. We become more focused, clear minded, and we feel less stress. Another study published in the Journal of Physical Activity and Health, shows that 20 minutes of yoga poses stimulate the brain more than walking or jogging for the same period of time.

d.Boosts the immune system

It is logical that as we improve our overall health, we improve our immune system as well. Actually, this is our only healing mechanism. The medications we take, the food supplements are just assistants and mostly soothe the symptoms of a disease. Our bodies themselves are retrieving their healthy condition through the immune system. So, daily practices can help our own healing system work properly and more effectively. Some scientists performed many studies and found evidence that yoga can enhance our immunity even on a cellular level. They also came to an interesting conclusion that practicing asanas regularly can even change our genetic expression! So, no more excuses such as *"I wasn't born flexible!"*, *"I have predisposition to gain weight!"*, *"I easily get ill!"*, etc. All these can be altered through healthy diet and some yoga!

e.Better sex!

Woohoo! That's what I'm talking about! Every time you exercise yoga, you increase your sexual potential. There are several ways in which yoga can improve your sex life.

First of all, obviously, you become more flexible. And this alone can make a huuuge difference – you know, all the poses you wanted to try, but never had the physical ability! Secondly, yoga helps us become more relaxed and more aware of our bodies. Most people have troubles in bed simply because of their anxiousness and lack of confidence. Another important point is that by doing asanas you get in touch with your own body and your senses become stronger. A simple touch of your partner can evoke stronger positive feelings. Finally, on a pure physical level, yoga stimulates the blood flow (especially to the genitals) and the secretion of hormones responsible for arousal. And this is equally valuable for men and women! Yoga practices have proven to be extremely helpful for females, because they strengthen the pelvic muscles. This not only gives them stronger and longer orgasms, but also makes them better equipped for easier child birth!

d. Improves your performance at work

"Why is it I always get my best ideas while shaving?" Albert Eistein

Some people can detest the exact same thing when they are in the shower or even more often – after a meditation. Experience has proven that when we feel relaxed and well rested we tend to be more productive, more creative, more efficient, and focused. This is one of the major reasons why many people turn to yoga and meditation. Yoga is not just physical poses, it should always end with breathing exercises and a short relaxation or visualization. It works holistically on our bodies and minds. Even business companies have embraced the idea of including yoga sessions throughout the working day for their employees, and soon results inevitably show up! Yoga and meditation has become quite popular among people of the corporate world not just because it's the current fashion, but because it has proven its benefits. The famous hedge fund founder, billionaire Ray Dalio says: *"Meditation, more than any other factor, has been the reason for what success I've had."*

e. Relaxes the body and mind

This is tightly related to the previous point. When we do yoga, we activate the parasympathetic nervous system. This part of the vegetative system is responsible for the expansion of the blood vessels, the dilation of the pupils, and the overall tranquility of the organism. Some people simply describe it with the phrase "rest and digest". One of the major tools, which our nervous system uses to accomplish its goal is hormone secretion, and more precisely – cortisol (the stress hormone), serotonin, and dopamine (the "happy" hormones). When we accumulate too much cortisol, the body feels distress – it may be experienced as high blood pressure, weak immune system, thyroid malfunction, slow metabolism, decreased muscle tonicity, etc. The good news is that yoga can prevent all these conditions just by decreasing our stress hormone levels! We become more relaxed, more centered, healthier, and happier!

Detoxing with yoga

Yoga stimulates the whole organism and all our organs. As it increases the blood and lymph flow, we help the body cleanse itself gently and easily. It is safe to say that each and every yoga session is beneficial and what we are looking for is the cumulative effect of persistence. Nevertheless, there are many asanas, which can facilitate the detoxing process in the body. Many people practicing yoga regularly notice how conscious they become about their bodies – what they eat and drink. As a consequence – making healthier diet choices becomes much easier and effortless. Some even experience a total repulsion from toxic foods and drinks, and others – naturally start intaking lighter vegetarian foods. So, here I will try to sum up some postures, which can help us get rid of the harmful agents.

a. Wide-Legged Forward Bend (Prasarita Padottanasana)

Execution:

Start by standing on your yoga mat with open feet (about 1 meter apart). If you are much taller, you may need to open the feet a bit more accordingly – with practice you will find the best distance. Make sure they are parallel to each other. Next, place your hands on your hips or your waist. Lift the arches of the feet a little bit as you press the feet on the floor to establish a strong stable foundation. Now, inhale and lift your chest and look up, but do not arch the torso, just keep your spine straight.

As you exhale lean forward using your hip joints. When your torso becomes parallel to the floor put your hands on the ground – they must be as wide apart as your shoulders and parallel to the feet. With both hands on the floor, fully expand your elbows and look up. Inhale. If you are not flexible enough to touch the floor, put a blanket or other helpful item on the ground to assist you until you are able to bend fully.

Next, as you exhale, lean down until your head reaches the ground. Roll your shoulder blades and stay in this position for 5 breaths. If you are a beginner, most likely you won't be able to touch the ground with your head. Do not despair or be discouraged! Just put some kind of suitable object below until the body responds to the pose.

Inhale and again expand the elbows and look up. Try to use the strength of your hips. Exhale and feel your feet as they press the ground. As you inhale go back up to your starting position.

Why is this pose valuable?

Practicing this asana regularly you will reap many benefits – you will strengthen the hips, legs and spine; it stimulates the brain activity while fighting harmful stress; it cleanses and tones the liver, the abdominal organs, and kidneys; relieves fatigue, mild cases of depression, and headaches.

b. Downward-facing dog (Adho Mukha Svanasana)

Execution:

Start by standing on your knees and hands on the mat. The hands must be pointing forward; you can spread the fingers a little bit. As you exhale start lifting your hips until they reach a 45 degree angle. Try to suck the belly and pull back the pubic bone. Your feet must be fully on the ground, but at first this may be difficult. In this case, stay on your toes and gently stretch the legs as you try to reach the floor, but do not press too hard – let the body adjust to the pose in time and with more practice. Also, keep the head down and relaxed, but not too loose. Try not to squeeze the shoulders tight and press the neck or to keep them slack – the spine must be straight.

Stay in this pose for a couple of minutes or as much as you feel comfortable to – one of the basic yoga principles is not to put too much pressure on the body and strain it.

Exit the pose as you exhale and bend the legs and place the knees on the floor.

Why is this pose valuable?

This posture is perfect for people working long hours sitting or standing still – it strengthens the upper back and stretches the spine. Among the many benefits of this asana are: relieves stress, headaches, fatigue, back pain, menopause and PMS symptoms. Tones the body, improves digestion, and prevents from osteoporosis, hypertension, sciatica, and sinusitis.

The pose is not recommended for pregnant women!

c. Plow pose (Halasana)

Execution:

Usually this pose starts from the pose Candle (Salamba Sarvangasana), but it is no problem if you start from lying on the ground. Place your hands on the mat beside the body facing down. You will use them as a support as you start lifting the legs above the ground. If it is still difficult for you to lift your legs, use your hands to support the spine (similar to the Sarvangasana pose). In case you are an absolute beginner and you still cannot lift your legs, try the place them against a wall. Use it as a support until you strengthen your core muscles. Continue until your toes touch the floor above your head. Your knees should be facing your forehead. Try to keep your back upward and perpendicular to the ground.

Usually the hands should be placed on the mat, but you can also lock your fingers on the floor. The chin should be pressing the breastbone.

Stay in the pose for a couple of breathes up to several minutes, or as long as you feel comfortable to.

Exit the pose by exhaling and slowly lifting the legs up and removing the toes from the floor. Use your hands to support the spine. As you lift the lower part of the body, here again you can stay in a Candle position for a few breaths. Exhale and slowly place your legs back on the mat. Give yourself some time to rest after the asana.

Why is this pose valuable?

This posture is extremely beneficial for the thyroid gland and the abdominal organs. It helps us reduce daily stress and fatigue. Doing Plow pose regularly can help people suffering from headaches, insomnia, sinusitis, and even infertility. It also relieves menopause symptoms; strengthens and stretches the spine and the upper body.

It is advisable for those who have severe back and neck injuries, diarrhea, asthma, or hypertension to avoid this asana. Also all inverted postures are not recommended during menstruation!

d.Staff pose (Dandasana)

Execution:

Start by sitting on the mat. Straighten the back and fully extend the legs (if you are able to). The legs should be together and the toes must be facing up. Stretch the spine as you push the sitting bone to the floor and point the top of the head (the crown) to the ceiling. Your back must be perpendicular to the ground, like a "staff". Your hands should be placed right beside the hips, the chest is lifted and shoulders are dropped down towards the back.

If you are not sure if your body is aligned, sit against a wall and check whether the only parts that touch it are the shoulder blades and the waist.

Why is this pose valuable?

This posture is valuable for it stretches and strengthens the back muscles, the shoulders and the chest. Although it looks simple, it can help you improve your posture tremendously. In case you have sciatica, Staff pose will be of great help for you.

Of course, if you have any injuries in your wrists or lower back, this asana may be counter indicated.

e. Sage's Pose (Marichiasana III)

Execution:

We start this asana from the previous posture – Staff pose. Sit straight on the mat with your legs in front of you and lengthen the spine (make sure it is perpendicular to the floor). Next, bend the right knee and place your foot on the ground. Now start gently twisting the body by placing the right hand behind you. Press the mat so that you stay stable. The left arm goes right in front of the right knee – the left elbow is touching the right knee, the arm is straight pointing the ground. The chest should be open, and neck twisted towards the right shoulder. You should be looking at the direction of the right shoulder.

Breathing in this posture is key – with each inhale lengthen the spine and with the exhale – twist the torso as much as you feel possible and comfortable.

You can stay in this pose for just a couple of breaths and with practice extend the time up to one minute. Remember to listen to your body!

Exit the pose by gently releasing the posture untwisting the spine.

Repeat on the other side: bend the left knee; put the left hand behind you and right one – in front of the bent leg.

Why is this pose valuable?

No matter how simple this posture looks, it should not be underestimated! It can give us great physical, mental, and emotional benefits. This asana gently massages the internal organs such as the kidneys and liver; improves digestion and fights constipation; stretches and strengthens the spine, the shoulders and lower back, and relieves pain in this area; it also stimulates the brain. Marichiasana III can help people suffering from chronic fatigue, sciatica, asthma, PMS and unpleasant menstrual symptoms.

This pose may not be suitable for those who have migraines, insomnia, diarrhea, irregular blood pressure (hypertension or hypotension), and spine injuries.

d.Revolved triangle pose (Parivrtta Trikonasana)

Execution:

Start by standing on the mat with your legs about a meter apart – the right foot is pointing straight forward, and the left one – at about 45-degree angle. As you establish this stable position, begin leaning forward from the hip joints. Raise your left hand and stretch down to reach the outer side of the right leg. At first it may be impossible for you to reach the ground. Do not worry – just use a suitable flat object on the floor to assist you until you gain more flexibility. Try to keep the torso straight, the chest lifted forward, and the belly – sucked in. Align the fingers of the left hand with the toes of the right foot. Press the mat for more stability. Next, raise the right arm upward keeping it perpendicular to the ground. The head is also turned upward – looking at the right arm. If it is difficult for you to face the ceiling, keep your head in a neutral position looking down or in front of you. Later on, as you progress, you will be able to fully perform the posture.

Again, stay in this position for as long as you feel it is natural for you. In time you will be able to hold it for up to a minute. Exit the pose by relaxing the raised arm down, untwisting the spine, and lifting the torso back to standing position.

Now, on the other side! Simply pivot the body to the left, keeping the same distance between the legs. The left leg must be pointing forward, while the right one – at 45-degree angle. Again, slowly lean forward and stretch your right arm to the ground. Don't forget to place the hand aligned with the toes of the left foot. Keep the back straight, the chest lifted, suck the tummy, and raise the left arm in the air pointing straight to the ceiling. Turn the head upward.

Why is this pose valuable?

This asana is a perfect example of an exercise that builds our stability, flexibility, and strength – in the legs, the hips, and the spine. This is a balancing pose which improves the work of the intestines, the lungs, and abdominal organs; improves breathing, and relieves back pains. People with sciatica, asthma, constipation, or other problems with the digestive tract will reap many benefits from this yoga pose.

Be aware, though, that Parivrtta Trikonasana is not recommended for those who suffer from chronic migraines, insomnia, severe diarrhea, and hypotension.

e. Seated Forward Bend (Paschimottanasana)
Execution:

Start this pose again from Staff pose – sitting on the mat with your back straight, the legs are stretched together, the feet are flexed (the toes are pointing upward). Now, inhale and stretch your arms over your head as you lengthen the spine. On the exhale, bend forward – try to bend from the hip joints instead of the lower back. Try to reach the feet with your hands. At first this may not be possible. But the goal is to stretch the spine as much as you feel comfortable and in time the body will be able to complete the pose. If you managed to reach the feet, grab the sides of the feet or put your index fingers around the big toes. If you are not able to do this, grab your legs as far as you can reach. To gently start stretching the spine in order to reach your toes, start lengthening the torso with each breath – on the inhale stretch the back, on the exhale try to move your torso slightly forward towards your feet. By doing this, with regular practice, eventually you will be able to complete the posture.

Keep you back straight and stay in the pose for at least half a minute or as long as you feel comfortable. In time you will be able to hold it for a couple of minutes.

Exit the pose on the exhale by releasing the posture and returning to the initial sitting position.

Why is this pose valuable?

This asana is perfect for increasing the flexibility and stretching the spine, the legs, hamstrings, and shoulders. This posture is also very beneficial for the internal organs – female ovaries and uterus, liver, and kidneys. In case you have hypertension, sinusitis, insomnia or infertility, practicing Paschimottanasana regularly can significantly relief these conditions. This asana is also applicable for the gastro enteric tract – it improves digestion, stimulates the appetite while increasing metabolism and fighting obesity. This posture is excellent for people who suffer from stress overload, depression, anxiety, menopause or menstrual discomforts. It relives the headaches, anxiety, and fatigue.

Although this asana is extremely helpful for many conditions, it has a couple of contraindications. If you have asthma, severe spine injuries or diarrhea, be careful while executing Paschimottanasana or avoid it altogether.

f. Locust Pose (Salabhasana)
Execution:
This asana is extremely valuable for the spine, but although it looks easy and simple, it could be rather challenging.

Start by lying down on your belly (prone position) and place your chin on the yoga mat, look straight ahead of yourself. Now place your hands beneath your thighs with your palms facing down – we will be using them as a support. Next, begin breathing slowly and deeply. On inhaling lift your legs off the ground with your toes pointing to the ceiling. Concentrate on your lower back and your butt – tighten the muscles in this area to maintain the posture. Hold your breath for as long as you feel comfortable. Now exit the pose by exhaling while slowly bringing the legs back to the ground. You can repeat the asana several times, if you wish.

Don't worry if you can barely lift your legs off the mat! This pose could take some time to master. If you want to prepare your muscles for this position, you can implement this asana with one leg at a time. In other words, lift your right leg while the other one is on the ground and hold for as long as you can. Then, do the other way around – lift the left leg and keep the right one on the mat. This way you will strengthen the lower back, the legs, and the butt. In time with some practice you will be able to lift up both legs.

Pay special attention to the breathing! It is very important, because it plays an important role in the healing process of yoga.

Why is this pose valuable?

This posture, if executed regularly, can significantly strengthen and stretch the abdomen, the legs, and lower back muscles. The posture also focuses on the buttocks, upper back, and lungs. Yoga poses such as this one can improve our overall posture. Practicing Salabhasana gently massages the internal organs, helping you improve your digestion and preventing from constipation. It could also be valuable for people having chronic back pain, or who are constantly gassy and bloated (flatulence). Yoga practices as a whole (asanas, breathing, and meditation) help us manage daily stress and fatigue. Nevertheless, there are some postures, which are extremely effective in energizing and toning our bodies when done regularly. Salabhasana is one of those power suppliers!

There are a couple of counter indications, though. Be careful with this pose if you have severe headache or any serious spine injuries.

g. Bow Pose (Dhanurasana)
Execution:

Lie prone on your yoga mat. Bend the knees and extend your arms towards them. Try to grab the upper part of the feet close to the toes. Place your chin on the floor for support. Try to relax the legs as much as possible. In case you cannot reach for the feet, use some kind of aid such as a strap. Use these additional tools until your body is flexible enough for you to grab the feet.

So, relax your feet and relax the buttocks – this is important for the proper implementation of the posture. This pose should not be executed from the muscles of the butt and thighs. Now inhale and as you inhale open the bow by lifting the chest and legs simultaneously. Your feet should be pointing up, look straight ahead of yourself. Try not to tighten the jaw muscles. Work with the pose as you are breathing – with each inhalation, extend the legs and chest, on the exhale try to keep your balance. Exit the pose on the exhale by relaxing the body into the initial position. Extend your legs and put your hands beside the body. Relax your head on the mat for some time.

If this pose was difficult to implement, try another version and see which one fits better for you. Or you can do them both. Start again lying prone on the floor. But this time hold your ankles instead of the toes. Put the chin on the mat and relax the legs on the buttocks. As you inhale lift the upper body (shoulders and head), and at the same time, pull with your shins backwards. In this variation the feet are flexed (not pointing up) and the thighs are not lifted from the ground. Look straight ahead. You can hold the position for half a minute or as long as you feel comfortable. Exit the pose on the exhale as you relax the body on the yoga mat. Rest for a little in supine position and repeat the posture once or twice.

Why is this pose valuable?

Dhanurasana focuses on strengthening and gently stretching the lower abdomen area, the hips, thighs, spine, upper back, neck, and breasts. This posture is beneficial for fighting fatigue, and discomfort in the back. People suffering from respiratory problems may have significant improvements from doing this pose. It also calms down the nervous system and relieves most menstrual symptoms. Just like every yoga pose, which focuses on strengthening the back muscles, this one improves the posture noticeably. Those who have frequent constipation should include Dhanurasana in their regular practices.

This pose also works beneficially for the internal abdominal organs.

Avoid this pose if you have very low or high blood pressure. People with chronic migraines or insomnia should also be cautious with this asana. Be careful executing Bow pose, if you have injuries in the spine (lower back or the neck). In case you experience pain or other negative sensations, exclude this pose from your routine.

h. Child's pose (Balasana)
Execution:
This is a very easy asana, excellent for ending your yoga routine, or making a tiny relaxation between other more challenging poses.

So, start by kneeling on the yoga mat. Extend your hands and place them on the floor in front of you.

Next, lean forward until your forehead reaches the ground. You will be sitting on your feet. Extend your arms fully and relax your body and mind. Breathe slowly and consciously. With each breath in, gently stretch the spine, and on the exhale, sink in between the thighs into deeper relaxation. You can stay in this position for as long as you wish or you can do a slight variation. Without moving your head and torso, bring your arms beside the body – palms are facing up. Again, relax the body, relax the shoulders, calm your mind, and breathe slowly. When you are ready, inhale, stretch the spine and lift your body up into your initial kneeling or sitting position.

Why is this pose valuable?

This posture is excellent for every yoga beginner. It is a must for everyone trying to relieve daily stress, and fatigue. It also works towards gently stretching the back muscles, the hips and thighs. Balasana is perfect for preparing the body and mind for entering a relaxed and meditative state.

This posture is not suitable for people with severe diarrhea, knee problems, and pregnant women.

i. Supported headstand (Salamba Sirsasana)
Execution:

Inverted poses are extremely beneficial for the body, especially for detoxification and rejuvenation. Nevertheless, this yoga posture could be very difficult for beginners. If you do not feel comfortable enough, don't do the pose on your own without an experienced yoga practitioner or instructor. But if you feel your upper body is strong and stable enough to perform this asana, you can start against a wall for support. You can also put some soft cushion below the head and arms for more comfort. Another excellent option for headstand beginners is to practice against the corner of the room. Both walls will further support the forearms and shoulders until they build more strength.

First, we will build the foundation of the pose. Sit on your legs on your yoga mat. Place your hands on the ground in front of you. To ensure the proper distance of the arms, wrap your hands on your elbows as you are kneeling on the mat. Next, without moving the elbows, just pivot the forearms and clasp your hands in front of you. Cup your hands - imagine as if you are trying to hold a sphere with them. Pay special attention to the little finger – tuck it inside the cup you made with your clinched hands, so you won't put too much pressure on it. Next, put the top of the head on the ground while the back of the head is wrapped inside the clasped hands. Press on the floor with the arms, the pressure and the main support of the body should be taken from the arms, not the head and neck. So press the arms on the mat and keep your shoulders straight. Be careful not to twist the forearms, keep them stable. Watch for and don't let the shoulders drop. Now flex your toes and lift the hips up so the body forms a triangle. Keep the spine straight, the butt is facing upward to the ceiling. Now start slowly walking towards the head, without crouching the back. Imagine as if the body is hanging on a string attached to the buttocks. Also pay some extra attention to the shoulders – they should be your main support. Press them to the floor without letting them collapse forward. As you keep this proper form, walk forward as much as you can. When you bring your legs as close as you can, try to slowly flex one leg in the air while the other is still touching the ground. Bring the knee as close to the chest as possible and squeeze it into the torso. Practice keeping your balance in this position for a couple of breaths. Now place the leg back on the mat, and flex the other one in the air. If you feel comfortable and the upper back is steady, try to slowly lift both legs in the air (one by one) without losing your balance. This part of the pose may take some practice to master. When you are ready, on exhalation continue with the pose and slowly extend the legs towards the ceiling. The toes should be pointing up. Hold this position for a couple of breaths, or as long as you feel comfortable. If you start to feel too much pressure on the neck, and it starts to drop down, this means it's time to come out of the pose. To reap the maximum benefit of the pose, you must stay in this position for at least 3-5 minutes. This won't happen overnight, it needs some practice and persistence.

Now it's time to exit the pose – start moving backwards. As you exhale, slowly bend the knees and bring the feet to the buttocks and try to keep your balance. Continue to bring the legs down as you engage the hip joints. When you touch the ground with the toes, come out of the pose completely as you sit on your legs.

Don't rush yourself to stand up immediately. Relax the body and normalize the blood flow by doing Child pose (see previous point) for a while. If you have put too much pressure on your upper body with Salamba Sirsasana, do some stretching of the neck and shoulders.

Why is this pose valuable?

Headstands are extremely beneficial for our bodies and minds. When executed regularly, Salamba Sirsasana can stimulate the organs in the abdominal area and thus, it can significantly improve our digestion. This pose strengthens the spinal and upper body muscles – arms, shoulders, back; builds strength in the core and legs. This posture, if done with proper breathing technique for a couple of minutes a day, can stimulate the lungs, and help people with asthma, or sinusitis. This asana relieves various uncomfortable issues, such as menopause symptoms, stress, insomnia, mild cases of depression. This headstand gently stimulates and strengthens the uterus, and significantly improves the chances of overcoming infertility. Last, but not least, this posture is extremely valuable for its beneficial effect upon our endocrine system. Salamba Sirsasana stimulates the hypophysis and the pineal gland in the human brain. These tiny glands are essential for the balance of the whole hormone secretion of the human body. For example the hypophysis (also called Pituitary gland) produces chemicals, which regulate and control important processes like: our metabolism, blood pressure, body temperature, the water balance in our organism, everything connected to procreation (the function of the genitals for both men and women, breast milk production, contractions of the uterus during childbirth, etc.), and assists the work of the Thyroid gland. The pineal gland is also affected beneficially from this posture. This part of our endocrine system is a little underestimated, because scientists haven't revealed its full potential. The Pineal is responsible for the secretion of the hormone Melatonin, which controls our so called 24-hour biological clock. If this gland works properly, we will have healthy refreshing sleep, less stress, and normal energy levels during the day. The Pineal gland also plays a significant role in our spirituality – its decalcification is considered to be the key to developing our intuition and clairvoyance (or clairaudience, clairsentience, etc.). It is a well-known fact that people, who practice yoga regularly, observe certain changes in their bodies, minds, and consciousness – they become more empathic, more intuitive, and more conscious about their diet and lifestyle.

Although this asana is extremely beneficial for our bodies and minds, it has some contraindications, which should not be overlooked. The first thing to consider, of course, is if you have any spine injuries, especially in the upper back and neck area. Be extremely careful with headstands (or avoid them completely) in case you have any heart diseases or irregular blood pressure – very low or very high. People with chronic headaches and migraines should also consider another yoga postures until they regain their health and wellbeing. All inverted poses (headstands, Candle, Plow pose, etc.) are not suitable for women during menstruation or pregnancy.

j. Chair Pose (Utkatasana)
Execution:

This pose (along with Child pose) is perfect for ending your daily yoga practice. This is a standing posture, so begin with standing upright on your yoga mat (keep your back straight). Place the feet right next to each other and spread the heels apart just a little bit (the toes are still touching). As the arms are resting down, turn the palms out and slightly bend the knees. Next, inhale and slowly continue to bend the knees while you bring the upper body forward. Imagine as if you are about to sit on a chair, don't forget to keep the back straight, do not arch the spine. Next, raise your arms straight upward – they should be aligned with the spine. You can lift the arms and bend the knees simultaneously or do it successively – the important thing is to keep a proper form. Press your feet on the ground for more stability. Pay attention to the shoulder blades – they must be down the back instead of shrugging. To test if you are holding the correct position, see if you are able so gaze at your toes. If not, you need to lean further forward. The full asana requires the hips to be parallel to the ground, but for beginners this will be difficult without putting too much strain on the lower back and knees. So, lower your body as much as it's comfortable for you without harming these areas. This posture should be felt mainly in the hips and quadriceps, instead of the lower back. Don't forget to draw in the belly and the tailbone down and forward (work with the hip joints) to keep the spine straight. When executing Utkatasana, also pay attention to the arms. They must be straight upward aligned with the spine, or you can press the palms together. But do not let the arms slack – engage the muscles of the arms and shoulders. For absolute beginners, this asana may be difficult at first. Chair pose requires strong leg muscles and some people may need a little support until they strengthen this body area. If this is the case for you, just practice the pose near a wall. When you lean forward to perform the posture, the tailbone should be touching the wall for support. Stay in this position as long as it feels comfortable and work your way up to one minute. Exit the pose with an inhale – straighten the knees as you lift your body from the arms muscles. On exhale, put the arms down beside the body (Mountain pose).

Why is this pose valuable?

Although this asana looks rather simplistic, it holds great value for our bodies. People who have flat feet will receive great benefit from practicing Chair pose regularly. This posture is also focused on strengthening the lower body – legs, hips, thighs, ankles. If executed properly, this asana will stretch the shoulders and chest, and will gently stimulate the heart, diaphragm, and the abdominal organs. The pose also engages the spine, especially the lower back area.

Be extremely cautious with this pose in case you suffer from chronic insomnia or headaches. Utkatasana is not the best choice for people with low blood pressure.

9. The Five Tibetan Rites

If you find the yoga poses in the previous chapter too challenging, do not despair. There is a yoga sequence of special movements, which can help you accumulate more vital energy and strength. They are called the Five Tibetan Rites. How do they connect with body detoxification? The link is not direct, but it could be sensed by anyone who started practicing them (or people who started doing yoga asanas regularly). The Tibetan Rites are actually a kind of a yoga practice, but they were specially developed for restoring our health, vitality, youthfulness, and stamina. For experienced yoga practitioners, these exercises may seem rather easy and simple, but they go beyond our physical wellbeing. I mention this yoga sequence here, because it's special – it influences the energy (chi) flow in our bodies and restores the balance in the chakras. Yoga practitioners know that there are seven main energetic points in our bodies called chakras. These chakras consist of constantly moving and rotating energy vortexes. When the individual is healthy and vibrant, these energy centers rotate with a normal speed and degree. When we become sick or when our bodies get older, the chakras slow down their rotation and the energy flow decreases. We feel less strength, less energy, and more and more fatigue.

If you are more "down to Earth" person and do not believe in such mambo-jumbo, I will explain briefly. Scientists and medical specialists confirmed that our bodies have several major points, which are highly wired with neurons (such as the Solar split). When we practice these special isometric exercises and breathe correctly (engaging the cardio-vascular system), we increase and stimulate the blood and lymph flow in these neuralgic areas, cleansing and healing them.

That's how the Five Tibetans became famous for their healing and rejuvenating properties. This yoga practice consists of simple daily rituals, which can help you restore your normal energy levels, your health, and youthfulness. Basically, these exercises are suitable for people of all ages. What you are going to need in order to receive all of their benefits is high concentration and focus, consciousness, and persistence.

This holistic yoga practice was developed by Tibetan monks for chakra balancing, restoring life energy in the body (chi), calming the mind and achieving meditative state more easily, slowing down the aging processes, and reducing stress.

People all over the world who started doing the Five Tibetan Rites detest all the beneficial effects they see in their lifestyle. In many cases regular practitioners of this yoga sequence observe higher energy levels, improved mood (and less mood swings), rejuvenation, weight loss, better vision and hearing, decreasing of chronic pains. It sounds too good to be true, but it all has a logical explanation. These special exercises, when done correctly with proper breathing, stimulate the blood and lymph flow. And as we know from previous chapters, when we improve the blood circulation, the toxins leave the body more easily through the natural cleansing system of the human   body.
From a physical perspective, this yoga practice is a form of exercising, which tones and strengthens the muscles. We also stretch and work with the joints, and thus

stimulate the secretion of synovial fluid (the natural joint grease) and the release of toxins accumulated in these areas. It has been proven from empirical evidence that regular practice of the Five Tibetan Rites improves our overall mental health – people become more energetic, calmer, less stressed, they sleep better, and have better memory.

How do these exercises actually work?

I have already mentioned about the connection between the Tibetan Rites and the chakras in our bodies. These are the keys to the health and rejuvenating effect of this yoga complex. There are seven main chakras located in different parts of our energetic bodies – the base of the spine, the navel, the solar plexus, the heart, the throat, at the center of the forehead, and the top of the head. These powerful energy and magnetic vortexes govern the flow of chi and the proper work of the endocrine system. The endocrine system is essential in every vital process – it is responsible for the complete and normal functioning of the human body, including the aging process. If we maintain our chakras in good shape, thus our hormonal secretion, we achieve better health and younger bodies. How do we take care of the energy vortexes? By maintaining their rotation speed high. That's what the Tibetan movements aim to do. The exercises are suitable for all ages, but remember to start slowly with a few repetitions, and always listen to your own body!

What therapeutic effects to expect when doing this yoga complex regularly?

I have already mentioned some of the amazing benefits of the "Tibetans". Let me summarize – these exercises improve our overall health. They are beneficial for the heart and lungs, improving our metabolism, digestion, and also strengthen the nervous system. When done regularly, this healing complex can relieve stress and back pain, balance the hormone secretion, vitalize and rejuvenate the organs, or even improve the eyesight.

Speaking about metabolism, we can conclude that the Tibetan Rites can have a slimming effect. When we achieve a balanced and correctly functioning endocrine system, it is much easier to have a healthy body weight. In case you are overweight, but you still want to implement these yoga exercises, be really careful. Do not push yourself too hard and begin with a few repetitions until you feel comfortable. When you master the Rites, slowly add more repetitions. If you feel any negative or painful symptoms, go back to fewer repetitions. The same rules apply for everyone, especially for the elderly. There are no age limitations, but pay attention and listen to your body. This is not a fitness program, it is an energetic work. In case you have any health conditions, make sure you consult with your physician before starting the Tibetans.

These yoga postures are not suitable for pregnant women, and people suffering from any heart diseases, hypertension, hernia, enlarged thyroid, severe cases of arthritis, and Parkinson's disease.

As for menstruation days, it depends on your personal reaction to this yoga complex. If you feel any discomfort, skip these days of the month, or do just a few repetitions.

The Five Tibetan Rites are also not recommended for pregnant women. Since these healing exercises are developed from male Tibetan monks, there is no original data about pregnancy. It depends on the personal decision of the mother-to-be whether to continue with the rituals or not. Make sure you consult with your doctor beforehand. If you decide to do the Rites during these months, be extremely careful. Do not push yourself, make fewer repetitions, and keep in mind that they could worsen the nausea in the first trimester. The last trimester is also very important, and it is best not to risk your pregnancy. Moreover, take into consideration that keeping balance with a big baby bump will be a hard task, and it could lead to dangerous traumas.

Breathing is key!

When executing the rituals, pay extra attention to the proper breathing technique. Our aim is to engage and stimulate the cardiovascular system, the blood and lymph flow. This is how the healing and cleansing effect is achieved. You can practice breathing even before starting the exercises. The technique is very similar to the ones described previously in the previous chapters. Since it is important to master it, it bears repeating.

Sit comfortably in a chair and straighten your back. Relax your shoulders, your chest, and mind. Place one hand on your abdomen and breathe in from the nose. Next, exhale through the mouth. On the inhale, you should feel the abdomen expand while the chest is stable.

This is abdominal breathing technique. Another exercise you can try before starting with the Tibetan Rites is full deep breathing. This time place one hand on the belly, and other one – on the chest. As you inhale, slowly expand the abdomen first and next – feel the air filling the lungs completely (the chest will expand, too). Exhale gently through the mouth or nose. Practice this pranayama (breathing yoga) for several minutes a day.

Another important tip before commencing the exercises is to execute them on an empty stomach. This will prevent you from feeling nauseous and the energy will flow more easily through the body.

Also try to do the Tibetans in the first half of the day. Even just a few repetitions can boost your energy and may cause insomnia.

Remember to start slowly. No matter how prepared physically you feel right now, start with 3 repetitions and observe any sensations (physical, mental, or even emotional) that may occur. Only when you feel completely ready increase the number with 1 or 2 more reps. In case you experience any discomforts, go back to fewer repetitions. These yoga exercises are not very difficult to perform from a physical perspective, but they can be extremely powerful energetically speaking. So, pace yourself, don't rush to reach 21 repetitions too quickly, and listen to your body! This may take a week, or months, or even a year, depending on your individuality.

Important note! People who have some serious issues and pains in the back and neck, for example – herniated disks, should be very careful when doing the Tibetan Rites. In case these exercises cause you any pain, I would recommend you start with the yoga postures first. You can use the asanas described in the previous chapter, or do a specific yoga sequence for the backbone. Feel free to consult and work with a yoga specialist, who can assist you with your healing process. After you have strengthened the back muscles, you can add to or substitute this practice with the Five Tibetans. Remember, you should not feel any pain, severe discomfort, or fatigue after exercising the Rites. Start small and you can always pause the practice or go back to fewer repetitions. Listen to your body! I know you are sick of me repeating this! :D

Shiva Shakti Mudra

This is another important breathing exercise that we will be using between some of the Tibetan rituals.

This is how you do it:

> Stand up with your back straight. The legs must be as wide apart as the shoulders. Slightly bend the knees. As you inhale deeply through the nose, start bending the elbows until they are parallel to the floor with your palms facing up. Imagine as if you are drawing energy from the ground upward.

> On the exhale (through the nose), roll your shoulder and push the energy forward until the arms are straight and parallel to the floor. Imagine as if you are pushing something away from you with both hands.

> Next, deeply inhale again and lift your arms upward at the 10 and 2 o'clock positions of the dial (the arms are forming the letter V).

> On the exhale, make semi circles with your arms with your palms facing towards your body. Slightly bend the elbows, so that both palms will meet each other in front of the genital area. But do not let your hands touch!

Let's get to the exercises:
1. Tibetan No. 1

Stand up straight with feet wide apart at shoulder level. Stretch the arms parallel to the floor. The left arm is pointing to the left, and the right arm – to the right. Turn one of the palms toward the ground, and the other – upward to the ceiling. Use your intuition to decide which palm to turn down and which one – up. Now, imagine energy entering your body from the palm, which is pointing up, and exiting through the palm, which is pointing down. You may feel the receiving hand warming, and the hand of giving – a bit colder. If you feel these sensations reversed, switch the hands' positions to match the energy flow. Next, start turning the body clockwise without moving the arms. Don't forget to start slowly with a few rotations (for example 3 times). Breathe slowly and consciously. If you feel dizzy from the rotations, choose an object from the room, and focus on it to avoid the nausea. After you finish with the rotations, inhale deeply, hold your breath, and exhale quickly and thoroughly. Bring your hands in front of the heart area in a prayer position.

This exercise looks very simple, but do not be fooled – it creates a swirl of energy, which accelerates the chakras and brings back their normal speed. This affects beneficially important organs, such as the liver, the thyroid, the master hormonal glands (pituitary and the pineal), the spleen, the reproductive system, and strengthens the knees.

2. Tibetan No. 2

Lie down on your back with legs straight and extend the arms alongside the body. Use your yoga mat for more comfort. The palms should be facing down. Now tighten the muscles in the abdominal and genital areas and exhale through the mouth. As you are exhaling lift your head until the chin reaches the torso. That's not all, while moving the head, lift the legs up as much as it's possible for you at the moment. Later you will be able to bring the feet over the head. Use the arms for support, but don't lift the pelvis, it should stay on the ground. Try to keep the legs together with knees straight. A quick recap of the exercise: on exhale you simultaneously lift the head and the legs, on inhale – the body goes back to starting position. Breathe deeply and consciously when executing these rituals.

Repeat 21 times or as many repetitions as you feel comfortable without feeling tired, and without panting.

This Tibetan concentrates on balancing the throat and sacral centers.

Before moving to the next exercise, do the Shiva Shakti Mudra breathing three times.

3. Tibetan No. 3

Kneel on the yoga mat with your back straight, and put your hands on the hips. Kneel on your toes in order to stimulate the reflex points on the feet, which represent the master glands – pineal and pituitary. On exhale (through the mouth), tilt your head forward (only the head do not move the torso) and press the chin on your chest (stimulating the Thyroid). Now inhale through the nose and lean back. Put your hands on the back of the thighs for support; tighten the muscles of the abdominal and genital areas; let your head drop backwards as you arch your back, bringing the abdomen forward. Exhale and bring the body forward and straighten the spine, press the chin to the breastbone. Note: on exhalation the spine is straight and you move only the neck and head forward. On inhalation, you arch the whole spine backwards.

Repeat the ritual as many times you feel comfortable and do the Shiva Shakti Mudra 3 times.

This exercise is extremely powerful stimulator for the reproductive organs. If you experience any problems in this area, this yoga ritual may even cause some dizziness. If so, do it with eyes open, and when you get used to the energy flow, start implementing it with eyes closed.

4. Tibetan No. 4

Start by sitting on the floor with your back straight and legs fully stretched forward. Next, place your hands on the ground right next to the pelvic area. If you remember the Staff pose from the previous point, this is the same posture. Start by exhaling through the mouth and tilt your head forward until the chin presses the chest. Now, tighten the abdominal and genital muscles and the neck, too. Inhale through the nose, and as you inhale without moving the hands, lift the pelvis upward and forward, step on the feet, move the head backwards. The body will form a rectangle. The back and the head must be aligned and horizontal to the floor. Exhale and bring the body back to the starting position with the chin pressing the chest. Repeat this procedure as many times as you can without feeling any negative sensations. This ritual may seem a bit harder, but with a little practice, it will get easier and easier.

Don't forget to perform the Shiva Shakti Mudra three times before continuing to the next exercise.

5. Tibetan No. 5

For those who practice yoga, this posture will be very familiar. Start by lying prone on your yoga mat. Place your hands on the floor at shoulder level. Turn your toes under, inhale through the nose, and push your body to form the Upward facing dog pose - the back is arched, the pelvis is relaxed, the head leans back, and the eyes are gazing upward. Don't forget to engage the abdominal and genital muscles. Keep the arms extended, but do not shrug them to the ears – keep the chest open. This will get easier with practice. On the exhale (through the mouth), lift the pelvis up so that your body forms a triangle, and press the chin to the chest. This is the Downward facing dog pose. Don't forget to keep the back straight, shoulders must not be tight around the neck (roll them down if necessary), and try to touch the ground with your heels. If this is not possible for you at the beginning, do not despair – in time the body will respond to the movement. On inhale, bring the body back to Upward facing dog, and so on. Repeat not more than 21 times.

This exercise, which combines these two basic yoga poses, is concentrated on stimulating the energy centers in the reproductive organs, the throat, and the brain. It strengthens the upper body, and the abdominal muscles; stretches the spine.

To properly finish this yoga sequence on an energetic level, lie down on your back. Now inhale and raise your arms above the head to stretch and enlarge the whole spine. Hold your breath in this stretched position for a couple of seconds, and exhale. As you breathe out, relax all the muscles of the body, and cover your face with your palms. Repeat this 3 times.

6. Tibetan No. 6

There is a sixth exercise in addition to the basic Five Rites. This ritual is not suitable and recommended for everyone. This special yoga sequence is created and applied mainly by Tibetan monks. And since they are celibate, they needed to channel their sexual energy in a positive, creative, and spiritual manner. Otherwise, the excessive sexual energy will create blockages. This is the purpose of the last Tibetan Rite. In other words, execute this ritual only if you consider that you have a strong libido, and you wish to channel this energy towards the higher chakras. If done correctly, it may even lead to developing psychic abilities, or feeling of deeper spiritual awareness and connectedness to the energy source. In other words, do this exercise only if you feel you have enough excess of sexual energy. If this is not the case, this ritual may do more harm than good. If your libido is low, just continue with the Five Tibetan Rites until your body reaches a balance of the energy flow, and every chakra is working properly.

This is the Sixth Rite itself: stand on your yoga mat with feet apart at shoulder level. Inhale slowly through the nose and completely fill your lungs with air. Then exhale through the mouth as quickly as possible. Now slightly bend the knees, lean forward and put your hands on top of the thighs. Try to exhale every remaining air from the lungs. Next, stand up and put your hands on the waist, but do not inhale. Hold it like this as long as you can. When you feel the urge to inhale, breathe in through the nose until you fill the lungs. Now exhale through the mouth and relax your hands gently hanging beside the body. Finally, breathe deeply in and out several times (through the nose or the mouth). Repeat this procedure three times.

Be persistent with the Five Tibetans to fully unlock their full benefit for the body, mind, and soul. Combining these rituals with more detoxing procedures, and healthier diet may completely transform your lifestyle, your health, your energy levels, and your self-esteem!

10.   Daily cleansing of the colon

It is no secret that nowadays we experience a lot of discomforts from the intestines - from constipation, through flatulence, even pain. Many people suffer from these types of colon problems, which means we need to help the intestines do their job. Our society has grown the habit of eating mainly processed foods, which clog the intestines and they cannot cleanse themselves properly. Specialists say we need to do the "number 2" at least once a day or even better – after each meal. If the bowel movement is too slow (once in a couple of days), this is a clear sign to pay extra attention to the colon. Don't forget the words of the father of Medicine, Hippocrates: *"All diseases begin in the gut."* Even if we go regularly to the toilet every day, we may have unexpected threats in this area. When food debris stay too long in the gut, they start to ferment and decay, creating toxic substances, which may be reabsorbed back into the bloodstream. Doesn't sound good, right? People with frequent constipation may experience regular headaches and skin issues, like acne or eczemas. Not to mention the overall poisoning of many organs and systems in the body. I don't mean to scare you, just to point out the importance of taking care of the colon. Don't freak out if occasionally under a lot of mental/emotional pressure you skip "number 2", especially when you are not in the comfort of your own home. But if this starts to happen too often, read on!

First of all, when we have such problems, we usually use the help of medications and/or food additives with strong laxative effect. This patches things up in the short term, but it has a detrimental effect on the long run. The body gets used to the medications and the external help for the bowel movement, and eventually the laxatives stop working. The walls of the colon deteriorate and stimulating them becomes harder and harder. This is why such medications (including some herbs) should be used sporadically for a short period of time, only for severe cases of constipation. The good news is that we can cleanse our gut, and have a regular bowel movement by simply changing our diet and/or our lifestyle. The price is not too high for the sake of our overall health and comfort. Remember to be patient, consistent, and to use the powerful force of synergy (combining two or more methods, which are suitable for your body and your lifestyle).

Here are some proven natural little steps you can try on a daily basis:

→ **A cup of hot water/tea for breakfast.** We have discussed this method previously, but it bears repeating. It looks so simple, but it's more powerful that meets the eye. Many people start their day with a hot cup of coffee, and usually it has a laxative and diuretic effect. Unfortunately, caffeine is not the best choice, because it irritates the stomach mucosa and can cause gastritis or even ulcers. What I found about the morning coffee, which stimulates the bowel movement, is not caffeine itself, but the high temperature of the beverage. Cold coffee does not have the same laxative effect. So, if you are a heavy coffee drinker, and you think that this drink helps you poop, think again. Next morning try with a nice hot cup of herbal tea. Try Peppermint/Spearmint, St. John's Wort, Oregano, Thyme, Melissa, dry Cranberries or Bearberries, Stinging Nettle, or any other option of your choice, personal taste and preference. Avoid using strong laxative teas for long periods of time, such as Senna, or Buckthorn. In the third book of the series (Build Your Immune System

Fast) , you will find a long list of herbs, which can be used with our cleansing regimen, with description of their healing properties, possible side effects, and dosages. Drinking hot tea (or water) in the morning can have an extremely beneficial effect – more than we expect. It cleanses all the food residues from the digestive tract, which had accumulated during the night; flushes out mucus and fatty substances from the walls of the stomach and intestines; improves the digestion; kills harmful microorganisms; dissolves slags and purifies the blood. As we know, if the intestines do not work properly and take out the food waste, it starts to ferment, produces toxic chemicals and gases, which easily enter the bloodstream. Just one cup of nice hot tea or water can successfully prevent this from happening. What else can we do on a daily basis that could gently stimulate the natural bowel movement and assist us with the cleansing process?

→ **Lemon juice and olive oil** – use freshly squeezed lemon juice and the same amount of extra virgin olive oil (1 Tbsp lemon juice and 1 Tbsp olive oil) to boost the work of one of the most important detox organ – the Liver Almighty. This simple cleansing procedure is done in the morning on an empty stomach. This is the perfect overture to the full liver & gallbladder detox ritual, which we will be discussed in the next book. But for now, just for the sake of beginning the cleansing process, this simple method is enough to stimulate the bile production. This ritual gently cleanses the bile ducts from stagnant bile, early stages of bile stones (grit), and other pathogenic debris. How is this connected to the regular bowel movement? The key is the bile, which has been produced in this process – it is a natural laxative. And also, don't forget how healthy lemon juice is. We talked about all the good stuff, which it brings to our bodies – huge amounts of Vitamin C, which cleanses and tones our bodies. On the other hand, extra virgin olive oil is a natural bile production stimulator and a joint and ligament lubricant with its large amounts of Omega-3 fatty acids.

→ **Flax seed beverage** – this morning drink is excellent for a healthy start of the day. It delivers large quantities of fiber, which stimulates the walls of the intestines, and cleanses them at the same time. It also contains lots of essential amino acids, the magical Omega-3 and Omega-6 fatty acids, and vitamin E, which are important for the cardiovascular system. Flax seeds are indispensable for people suffering from hypertension and problems with irregular bowel movement. So, how to prepare this morning health bomb? It is extremely easy: just mix 1-2 Tbsps. freshly ground flax seeds with a cup of water and stir. If you prefer something sweet, just add some honey. Just remember that the water's temperature must not be higher than the human body temperature, in order to preserve the vitamins and microelements in the honey. To get the maximum benefit from the flax seeds' healthy compounds, grind the seeds just before ingesting them. In this way you will prevent its compounds to die out. Another helpful tip: after drinking this beverage, try to take one more glass of water – the flax seeds absorb large quantities of liquid, and thus it starts to swell and enlarge its volume – this helps with the better stimulation of the intestine walls.

➜ **Fruit breakfast** – this is the perfect breakfast for everyone, but for people with lazy bowels, fruits are a must. They supply us with lots of fiber, which gently cleanses the intestines and flushes food debris, mucus, and other "trash" out of our bodies. These sweet and colorful products of Mother Nature are packed with essential vitamins, microelements, enzymes, charging us with energy, toning and hydrating us. It is important to know that not all fruits are made equal. Some have extremely costive effects (quince, pomegranate, cornels, cherries and sour cherries), but others are famous with their gentle laxative properties (watermelon, melon, plums, apples, grapes, etc.).

➜ **Leafy greens (salad or smoothie)** – fresh green vegetables or smoothie made from them is the ultimate detox and anti-constipation natural tool. But you can go even further – consider taking seedlings as a salad additive or a smoothie. They may look just like a normal vegetable leaf, but don't be fooled. Seedlings are powerful nutrition and healing sources. Take a look at all the benefits of the juice extracted from these magical small plants:

    ✓ Packed with Vitamin A and C;

    ✓ Contains easy absorbing Vitamins from group B, including B17 (called laetrile), which has shown acute anti-cancer properties without harming the normal body cells;

- ✓ Seedlings juice is a natural source of Calcium, Phosphorus, Magnesium, Sodium, and Potassium in a well-balanced ratio;
- ✓ Supplies with the essential Iron, indispensable for the blood cells formation;
- ✓ Contains more than 90 microelements, essential for our wellbeing;
- ✓ A perfect assistant in your Chlorophyll therapy – the chlorophyll's molecule is very similar to the hemoglobin. This means that natural chlorophyll sources help us with the oxygen transportation through the blood stream. Subsequently, this proper oxygen supply cleanses our bodies from toxic accumulations, activates the lymph system and accelerates the healing processes;
- ✓ Lowers the high blood pressure;
- ✓ Cleanses and assist the liver;
- ✓ Prevents from the formation and accumulation of metabolic toxins (the waste, which our cells produce);
- ✓ Helps with regulating normal blood sugar levels;
- ✓ Many people consuming fresh leafy greens (especially seedlings) report that their hair starts to reverse the graying and hair loss process;
- ✓ Prevents from and heals constipation;
- ✓ Builds resistance and counteracts the symptoms from radiation;

✓ Has strong antiseptic properties and kills harmful bacteria in the blood, lymph, and tissues;

✓ Contains all essential amino acids for the human body, and many more.

→ **Sprouts** – daily consumption of sprouted seeds can heal all kinds of physical conditions and bring back the normal bowel movement. There is a huge difference between a normal seed and a germinated one. In the sprouting process a lot of enzymatic processes are activated, and the seed starts to accumulate many biologically active compounds. These compounds are essential for our healthy nutrition. For example, a sprouted wheat seed has 1.5 times more Vitamin B1, 13.5 times more Vitamin B2, 5 times more Vitamin B6, 4 times more Folic acid, and 5 times more Vitamin C. The same accumulating process applies for other essential vitamins (Vitamin A and E). Don't worry about overdosing with sprouts; this super food contains natural antagonistic connection between some vitamins. As an example, large quantities of Vitamin B1 and PP can damage the liver, but germinated seeds contain choline, which neutralizes them. Sprouts are not only full of vitamins, they also have lots of microelements and fiber, which makes them a perfect natural additive for daily cleansing the colon, and healing constipation. All the above mentioned beneficial compounds found in these small seeds can be powerful assistants in fighting even the most serious illnesses, such as cancer, diabetes, anemia, chronic infections, infertility, intoxication, weakened eyesight, chronic fatigue, radiation, female reproductive hormone imbalance, etc.

How to make your own sprouts at home? It is not that difficult. First of all, choose your seeds – they could be any type as long as they haven't been treated with chemicals and/or high temperatures. They also need to have their coat intact. It is best to choose your seeds from a trusted bio store and brands – you will be sure the seeds will be high quality and GMO free. Start the germinating process by soaking the seeds in a container filled with pure water. Avoid using tap water, unless you are sure it's clean. This soaking procedure dissolves the inhibitor compounds in the seeds, which suppress the germinating process. Let them sit for a couple of hours, and rinse them thoroughly. Next, put the seeds in a container with a lid. It is best to use a glass jar instead of plastic containers. Spread them on the bottom, seal the jar, and put it in a dark place (the cupboard, for example). Keep the seeds always moist and rinse them thoroughly at least twice a day. Most seeds need between a day or two to germinate. The optimal root length is 1.5 - 2 mm. If you leave the sprouts to develop further, you will have nice, healthy, green seedlings. As we mentioned in the previous point, only the green parts of the seedling are good for consumption. One important note regarding sprouts: some seeds form mucus during germination. These are flax seeds, watercress, rocket salad, mustard seeds, etc. For these types of seeds it is best to put cheesecloth beneath them in the jar.

This way it will be much easier to rinse them well during the process. Another important thing to consider is the legumes sprouts – most of them (especially beans) contain a compound, which is not good for us. It is called phytohaemagglutinin. This chemical is the reason why we cook beans longer and even throw away the "first water", in which they were cooked. Phytohaemagglutinin can be found in even larger quantities in bean sprouts, so if you decide to germinate these seeds, you need to bake or boil them for several minutes (10 minutes at best). If you want to stay 100% raw, it is a good idea to avoid bean sprouts.

Always rinse the sprouts thoroughly with clean water before consuming them.

→ **Ground raw sesame** – just like the flax seeds drink, which I mentioned previously, ground sesame is full of natural fiber, and thus helps us with the normal and regular bowel movement. But that's not all! Sesame holds more power in its tiny seeds than meets the eye! It is packed with goodies – it contains lots of Magnesium, Copper, and Calcium. One cup of these seeds (about 30-40 grams) supplies us with around 75% of our daily need of Copper, 35% - of Calcium, 32% - of Magnesium, 29% - of Iron, and 18% - of Zinc. I think I don't need to explain how important these microelements are for a balanced and a healthy lifestyle. Sesame has much more to offer, especially for the ladies! It supplies us with many antioxidants, which slow down the aging process; also a phytoestrogen called sesamine, which balances the female hormones, prevents from osteoporosis, and fights cancer. Sesame seeds or raw sesame tahini are extremely beneficial for people with osteoporosis, anemia, cardiovascular issues, all pregnant, breastfeeding, and menopausal women, athletes, or people exposed to physical or mental stress. These tiny seeds help us have stronger hair and nails, enhance our eyesight and hearing, boost the quality and quantity of the sperm, heal and prevent constipation and even cough. Everyone who suffers from hypertension, chronic fatigue, hyper sweating, or hyperactivity should consider including sesame in their diet.

→ **The pose** – you may be surprised, but when we talk about colon cleansing, bowel movement, and constipation, the pose, in which we defecate, is extremely important. We have always been taking "the number 2" in squatting position, unlike nowadays when we normally defecate sitting, due to the invention of the modern toilet seat. When we take a look at the anatomy of the colon, we see the rectum at the end of the anal canal. When it's time to evacuate the colon, but we are standing, lying, or sitting, the rectum is automatically tightened so that the feces stay in place until we find a place to defecate. The only time the anal canal naturally loosens up completely in order to fully evacuate our organic waste is when we squat. Unfortunately, since the toilet seat spread around the world, most people defecate in a sitting position, which does not allow the rectum to open up to its full capacity. The result is not very pleasant - we cannot evacuate the colon completely and feces debris may remain in the intestines, which slowly infiltrate our system. On the other hand, since this evacuating process is incomplete, we are usually forced to push hard to take out all the waste. The result is painful and uncomfortable – hemorrhoids, diverticulosis, appendicitis, and other various intestinal infections. A quick recap – if you frequently struggle with constipation, defecate hardily with a lot of effort, if you have hemorrhoids, or if you often have the feeling of incomplete feces evacuation, keep in mind that the cause may be the unnatural defecation position.

What is the solution? There are some easy adjustments you can try in order to help with the process. You can put a stable object under your feet, so that the torso and the legs maintain about 35-degree angle. Special squatting stands are gaining more and more popularity. Some of these products enable you to fully emulate the natural squatting defecation position. Some people take this issue very seriously and even build floor squatting toilets (also called Indian or Turkish toilets) in their homes. They may be more inconvenient without letting you sit comfortably on a seat and browse the web with your phone, but they are surely healthier. If you are willing to give this method a try, choose the easiest option for you, and observe the results!

➔ **Movement** – we are back on the exercise topic, but this is something we tend to neglect in our hectic and busy lifestyle. There are many health authors who state that constipation can be eliminated simply by increasing the water consumption and physical activity. As we already know, sweating is an excellent easy technique to get in shape, strengthen the immune system, disease prevention, lose some extra pounds, detox, and as it turns out – it helps you poop, too. Choose a form of activity, which gives you joy, that's how you will get the motivation to continue. It could be anything – dancing, aerobics, biking, football, Pilates, or my personal favorite – yoga. I keep focusing on yoga, because it keeps proving itself to be extremely effective, especially nowadays when we sit on the computer more than we should. I will share with you some easy postures, which promote the natural bowel movement. Another good thing about yoga is that it doesn't take much time to do a couple of poses. Here they are:

a. ***Plow pose (Halasana)*** – you already know this pose from the previous chapters, but you don't need to scroll back to find it. If you missed it, here it is one more time:

Execution:

Usually this pose starts from the pose Candle (Salamba Sarvangasana), but it is no problem if you start from lying on the ground. Place your hands on the mat beside the body facing down. You will use them as a support as you start lifting the legs above the ground. If it is still difficult for you to lift your legs, use your hands to support the spine (similar to the Sarvangasana pose). In case you are an absolute beginner and you still cannot lift your legs, try the pose against a wall. Use it as a support until you strengthen your core muscles. Continue until your toes touch the floor above your head. Your knees should be facing your forehead. Try to keep your back upward and perpendicular to the ground.

Usually the hands should be placed on the mat, but if you can, lock your fingers on the floor.

Stay in the pose for a couple of breathes up to several minutes as long as you feel comfortable to.

Exit the pose by exhaling and slowly lifting the legs up and removing the toes from the floor. Use your hands to support the spine. As you lift the lower part of the body, here again you can stay in Candle position for a few breaths. Exhale and place your legs back on the mat. Give yourself some time to rest after the asana.

Why is this pose valuable?

This posture is extremely beneficial for the thyroid gland and the abdominal organs. It helps us reduce daily stress and fatigue. Doing Plow pose regularly can help people suffering from headaches, insomnia, sinusitis, and even infertility. It also relieves menopause symptoms; strengthens and stretches the spine and the upper body.

It is advisable for those who have severe back and neck injuries, diarrhea, asthma, or hypertension to avoid this asana. Also all inverted postures are not recommended during menstruation!

b. The gas releasing pose (Pawanmuktasana)

Execution:

Start by lying on your back on the yoga mat. As you inhale, raise one of your legs (for example the right one) and bend the knee. Raise your upper body at the same time, hold your leg with both arms and try to touch your knee with your nose or the chin. Try not to lift the other leg from the ground. Breathe evenly and hold this position as long as you feel comfortable to. On exhale return your body to exiting position (lying supine). Next, repeat the same procedure with the other leg. Next, we are going to do the same posture by lifting both legs. Inhale, bend both knees, lift the upper body, hold your legs and try to touch the knees with your nose/chin. The legs must be tight together; you can also embrace your legs by clasping the opposite elbows. Again, stay in this position as long as you feel good and breathe normally. Exhale and go back to lying supine on the yoga mat. When you get used to this pose, you can try one interesting variation. Inhale and lift one of your legs again and bend the knee again. This time you will need to lift the leg a bit higher so that you will be able to grab your heel/foot with both hands as you touch the knee with your nose/chin. You may already suspect what's next – breathe naturally as you stay in this pose, then on exhaling bring back the body back to starting position, and repeat with the other leg. This variation (just like the first one) can be done with both legs bent. The breathing pattern is the same. When holding the pose, try to relax the body. Do not strain or stretch the muscles of the neck and thighs too much. If you have strong pains in the neck, or any kind of injury you can hold the head on the ground while executing the asana.

Why is this pose valuable?

This yoga pose is focused on the lower areas of the body – strengthening and stretching the muscles of the legs, the butt, hips and thighs, relaxes the abdomen. It also stretches the back and neck; this asana works as a gentle internal organ massage – it improves the blood circulation in this area, improves digestion, evacuates the accumulated gas, fights constipation, supports the reproductive organs (counteracts infertility, sterility, impotence, and menstrual imbalances). This pose is excellent for strengthening the belly muscles and shredding fat from this area.

Pawanmuktasana should be avoided from people, who suffer from hernia, or hemorrhoids, and those who underwent a recent abdominal surgery. This pose is also not suitable for pregnant women.

c. *Half Spinal Twist (Ardha Matsyendrasana)*

Execution:

Sit up on the yoga mat with your legs extended in front of you and back straight. Next, lift the left leg, bending the knee, and bring it over the right leg. This means the left foot steps on the outer side next to the right leg. Bring the left leg as close to your torso as possible, without losing balance. Now extend the left arm, slightly twist the torso, and place the left hand behind you. Bend the right elbow, place it on the left side of the left knee, and press gently to the right so that the torso twists further. Try to keep the legs fixed and focus on twisting the spine. Exhale and return to the starting position. Repeat on the other side.

Why is this pose valuable?

This pose is excellent for stretching and strengthening the spine, the back, and the neck. It stimulates the digestive system, supports the liver, and the kidneys. It also works wonders for overcoming stiffness in the hips and shoulders. This spinal twist is good for the reproductive system, too – it relieves menstrual discomforts and prevents from infertility. People with asthma, sciatica, and chronic fatigue may also find great benefit from this asana.

Avoid this pose or work with a yoga master if you have any spine or back injuries.

d. *Raised Legs Pose (Utthanpadasana)*

This pose is focused on strengthening our core muscles, and thus – helps us increase the blood flow in the abdomen. This heals and prevents from discomforts connected to the intestines, including constipation.

Execution:

Start by lying supine on the yoga mat with your arms beside the body. Inhale deeply and as you breathe in start lifting one leg. Lift as high as you feel comfortable. Try to keep both legs straight in the process. Hold this position for a couple of seconds and release slowly while exhaling. Repeat the same procedure with the other leg. You can make several repetitions. Next, we are going to do the same exercise with both legs. Again, inhale slowly and start lifting both legs without bending the knees. Try to keep the core muscles tight throughout the whole sequence.

Why is this pose valuable?

First of all, as I already mentioned, this pose is excellent for toning the abs, especially the lower abdomen. The digestive and reproductive systems also benefit from this asana. Utthanpadasana strengthens and stretches the hips and thighs. It is excellent for recovering the strength and elasticity of the genital muscles after childbirth or recovering from a prolapse. Last, but not least – by strengthening the core and increasing the blood flow in this area, we easily get rid of excess fat tissue.

A few words of caution: do not execute this asana if you have high blood pressure, peptic ulcers, abdominal hernia, or if you had undergone any kind of surgery in this area. This posture is also not suitable for pregnant women, and during menstruation.

e. *Butterfly pose (Badhakonasana)*

This is an excellent and gentle pose for the lower body.

Execution:

Sit on the yoga mat. You can put a pillow or a blanket beneath you in case you feel uncomfortable. Next, bend the knees and bring the legs closer to the body. Now let the legs go down on both sides and let the soles of the feet touch each other. The legs now look like two wings of a butterfly. Next, as the feet press each other, try to slowly and gently reach the ground with your knees. At the beginning this may not be possible, and be careful not to strain yourself. Next, grab the feet and hold tight. On inhale, start to slowly lift the legs while the feet are anchored on the floor. On exhale, bring the legs down until they reach the ground (or as low as you feel comfortable). The movement resembles the flapping of the butterfly's wings. When you get a handle of this process, you can accelerate to a comfortable speed. Next, slow down the movement and eventually stop.

Now inhale deeply and on the exhale, press the tailbone and the feet to the ground and slowly bend forward. Keep your gaze in front of you and the spine straight. Move your elbows on your thighs or knees and push the legs towards the floor. Breathe deeply and consciously, with each breath relax the muscles of the legs further and bring them closer to the ground. Breathe in and release the pose.

Why is this pose valuable?

This yoga pose is concentrating on the lower body – it is a gentle, but effective hip opener. Badhakonasana stretches the thighs, increases the flexibility and the blood flow of the genital area and the hips. It promotes the regular bowel movement and prevents from constipation and other gut issues. Relieves the menstrual discomfort and tiredness of the legs and feet. This pose is suitable and even extremely beneficial for pregnant women – if practiced regularly, it assists with the natural childbirth process.

→ **Stress and constipation** – at a first glance there is no obvious connection between them, but that's not true. Our mood, the daily stress, which we experience, the emotional and psychological state, in which we are, even our thought patterns affect our gut health (and our overall health of course). We often forget that our intestines are called "our second brain". We experience most of our emotions in this area – tightness in the stomach, "butterflies" in the tummy, etc. It has been proven that stress, anxiety, and depression are the main culprits, or the "unlocking" factors for most digestive problems – gastritis, ulcers, colitis, IBS, and so on. This also applies for our bowel movement. The more sensitive and delicate person you are, the more stress affects your "pooping". Just think about how many people are unable to do "number 2" in unfamiliar environment (outside their homes), or if there are other people around. This is purely a psychological barrier. Unfortunately, we have more of these stress factors without even realizing it, such as chronic negative thinking patterns. The New Thought movement, especially Louise Hay, explains how frequent constipation may be a result of our refusal of old ideas, or holding too much to the past. You have probably heard phrases like *"Back in the day things were better!"*, *"The new generations are far worse!"*, and so on. So, if you have changed your diet, you exercise, you drink enough water, and still suffer from frequent constipation, maybe the key here is in your own head. Release all the stress in any way you can (earlier in the book we talked about breathing and yoga, they can do an excellent job), take notice of the negativity from the past you need to release. Maybe you need to forgive someone, or just looking at your life in a more positive and optimistic manner. If you are a fan of the New Age principles, you can add some supporting daily affirmations, or do some relaxing meditation or visualization. Here is a sample affirmation for constipation from the affirmation guru Louise Hay: *"As I release the past, the new and fresh and vital enter. I allow life to flow through me. It is safe to experience new ideas and new ways.*"

Final words

Remember that synergy, persistence, and consistency are key. Try to devise your own daily detox ritual that fits your lifestyle and preferences. For example, wake up earlier, drink some natural lemonade, do some cardio and sweat out even more unnecessary chemicals. Combining this ritual with gradually elimination of most common toxins and you are on the path to a cleansed, healthier, and more energetic body! You may not have to start with long deep cleansing procedures right away. Keeping optimum health and weight is an ongoing process, rather than a three-day wonder. Slowly building new healthier habits is easier and will have more long lasting beneficial effects. Pick your favorites and experiment. And when you feel ready to upgrade, you can dive deeper into the detoxing processes, which will be described in the next book.

Thank you!

I want to thank you for purchasing this book and reading it all the way to the end. I hope it has been helpful and informative. If you liked this volume, you can support my work and make it more visible for others who are looking for this kind of knowledge! I would deeply appreciate if you take a minute and write a short review on Amazon. I thank you in advance for your support!
Kind regards and best wishes,
Milica

P.S. And don't forget to get your free ebooks:
"10 Powerful Immune Boosting Recipes"
"12 Healthy Dessert Recipes"
"15 Delicious & Healthy Smoothies"
"The Complete Ayurveda Detox"

Go to *www.MindBodyAndSpiritWellbeing.com* and claim your gifts!

Or simply scan the QR code below:

About the author

Milica Vladova dedicated her work to spread the valuable knowledge of the physical, emotional, and spiritual wellbeing. She is determined to make the world healthier, happier, and more successful!

Her works have been published on *The Huffington Post*, *Thrive Global*, *Steven Aitchison*, and more.

Find her on:
http://mindbodyandspiritwellbeing.com
https://facebook.com/**mindbodyandspiritwellbeing**
https://www.pinterest.com/**milicavladova**
https://twitter.com/**Holistic_Milky**

Milica is also the author of:

Complete Body Cleansing and Strong Immunity Bundle

- **Healthy recipes** with white sugar and white flour alternatives!
- Plenty of toning, refreshing, and cleansing **smoothie recipes**!
- Detoxing and strengthening aromatic **herbal blends**!
- Loads of delicious **immune boosting recipes** and remedies.
- Which exercises can help us **expel more toxins** from our cells;
- **Simple weekly, monthly, and annual detox rituals** to help you boost your energy, lose weight naturally, fight chronic fatigue, and prevent from diseases.
- How to purify your system **without starving**?
- How to **deeply detox and heal your colon, liver, kidneys, lungs, lymph**, and more?
- How to naturally **get rid of parasites**?
- **Healthy gut - healthy you!** How to take care of our beneficial colon bacteria?
- **Natural probiotics and prebiotics** - how to make them at home with natural ingredients?
- **Adaptogens** - the key to dealing with stress, infertility and building our strong immunity.
- Natural ways and systems to **prevent, stop, and heal from cancer** cell formation.
- **The best herbs, essential oils and homeopathic remedies** to prevent from diseases, viruses, fungi, and bacteria.
- and much more!

★★★★★Science mixed with love for a winning combo

What a wealth of information filled with knowledge and innate insight into how the body functions and heals. So many great choices offered. These books are wonderful at dipping into every day for fresh ideas. Just applying some of the knowledge is still so powerful at helping you get fit and healthy from the inside out. Great recipes and full of science mixed with genuine love from the author.

~ **Reviewer on Amazon.com**

★★★★★Accessible, clear, and gently written

I wish all health books were written this way!

First, Ms. Vladova shares exhaustive information on cleansing and eating well with such a gentle, non-judgemental attitude.

And she meets the reader where they are. For instance, after introducing the Weekly Fasting Day with just tea or Water, Ms. Vladova suggest that if that is too extreme for you at the beginning, you can start with a day of fasting that involves Green Smoothies instead. And if even that is too much, she offers a plan for a day with just rice and apples.

As someone who's never tried any cleanses, her approach was so accessible!

Second, there is NO FLUFF! She gets right into talking about how to eat better and cleanse your body.

Recipes are easy to understand and well explained.

~ **J D on Amazon.com**

★★★★★ **The Perfect Christmas Stocking Filler - A Recovery Programme for those who Overindulge**

Gosh, this is a must-buy for anyone who cares about their body.

I'd already had some great results from the Healthy Body Cleanse detox programme, but the other two books are an absolute bargain - so full of useful information to keep you on track.

Although it's a great Christmas pressie for those of us who have no willpower in the season of gross overindulgence, it's actually a great regime to follow in the month before to prepare your body for the onslaught.

A win-win either way.

~ FireDancer on Amazon.com

★★★★★**A great resource!**

What a wonderful resource, so jam-packed with information! The body has a great mechanism to heal itself and these books help with that. I'm really pleased because my daily smoothies are now more interesting with the recipes included. The other recipes are easily adapted if you are vegan like I am. This bundle is what I would term a coffee-table book because once you've read it through you can dip into it every day or whenever you need to be reminded of the great info inside. My health has greatly improved and I recommend this bundle to anyone on the same journey to health or thinking about it.

~ Karen Aminadra on Amazon.com

DIY Homemade Beauty Products Bundle

MORE THAN 500 NATURAL ORGANIC BEAUTY RECIPES FOR THE WHOLE BODY!

What are you going to find in this book?
- Universal **face masks** for all skin types.
- **Lotions and cremes** for oily, dry, and mature skin.
- **Anti-aging and rejuvenating serums** for the face and eye contour.
- Natural **remedies for acne, pimples, blackheads**, etc.
- Gentle **whitening treatments** for brighter complexion and radiant skin.
- Universal nourishing **hair masks**;
- **Hair repair** recipes;
- **Anti-split ends** treatments;
- Natural **remedies for hair-loss** and thinning hair;
- **Hair growth** stimulators;
- **Dandruff healing masks** and ointments for oily and itchy scalp;
- **Herbal rinsing, organic shampoo recipes** and oil blends;
- Nourishing **body butters and lotions**;
- **Non-toxic sunscreen** recipes;
- Cleansing and healing **body scrubs and exfoliators**;
- **Anti-cellulite treatments** and massaging oils;
- Nourishing and **anti-aging hand cremes** and masks;
- **Nail strengthening** procedures;
- Natural **toothpastes and mouthwashes**;

- and more...

★★★★★Great deal!

This budle is a great resource for homemade beauty products! These are gentle and natural products!

~ **Kelly Phister on Amazon.com**

★★★★★Great set of books that has numerous recipes for everyone

Great set of books that has numerous recipes for every item.

The ingredients required are not difficult to come by. Overall a very nice and helpful set of books that comes in very handy for lotions and hand creams, hair masks etc. I recommend this book.

~ **Joanne Beal on Amazon.com**

★★★★★Start saving money and be healthier, too!

Talk about your natural resource for all things you purchase. Now I am the first one to tell people to stop buying prepare items like soap, shampoo and the like, and to make their own. I go to Lush religiously and purchase their items. It is all natural barring a few essential ingredients that are needed to preserve the products, and even them it is as gentle and natural as possible. Show yourself some love and get this book, and save yourself some money at Lush, because their products are not cheap and this DIY boom is loaded with so much and really is worth the small price investment as you will save literally thousands with all these recipes and all the imformation!

~ **Aisha Hashmi on Amazon.com**

The Healthy Vegan Recipes Cookbook

MORE THAN 80 HEALTHY VEGAN RECIPES FOR THE WHOLE FAMILY!

 In this volume you will find:
- Healthy vegan **main course dishes**;
- **Bread and salty snacks** recipes.
- **Dips and side dishes.**
- Yummy **sugar-free desserts.**
- Interesting info about **the numerous benefits of vegan foods.** and more!

★★★★★**Perfect when you're in a pinch!**

I referred to this recipe book several times over the past week to get some healthy, tasty recipes for my vegan/vegetarian friends. The author definitely has first-hand experience preparing these dishes, provides clear tips and alternatives, and also imparts knowledge about the health benefits. I'm short, it's a practical recipe book, but it's also an insightful read. I'll be reaching for this book over the holiday season for more inspiration. I'm thinking of pulling together a raw nut loaf and I'm pretty sure I saw a recipe in here I could swing! I know it won't disappoint! (I'm considering purchasing a hard copy this Xmas for a raw food friend!)
~ **Cynthia Luna on Amazon.com**

★★★★★**Try these recipes!**

Lots of wonderful recipes that I cannot wait to try. Healthy and nutritious meals! Snacks!
~ **Aisha Hashmi on Amazon.com**

Printed in Great Britain
by Amazon